The Uncertain Miracle

PERMISSIONS

I am grateful to the following publishers, authors, and organizations for permission to quote from the works named below:

Proceedings of the Third International Conference of Hyperbaric Medicine, ed. Ivan W. Brown Jr., MD., and Barbara Cox. (1966) Reprinted with permission of the publisher, The National Academy of Sciences.

Hyperbolic Oxygenation and Its Clinical Value, Dr. N. G. Meijne, copyright1970 by Charles C. Thomas. Reprinted by permission of. Charles C. Thomas and the author.

"The Compressed Air Bath and Its Uses in The Treatment of Disease," Dr. C. Theodore Williams, British Medical Journal, April 18, 1885. Reprinted by permission of British Medical Journal.

"Everybody's Business—What's Next in Science" by Floyd W. Parsons, The Saturday Evening Post, March 5, 1921. Reprinted by permission of The Saturday Evening Post.

"The Cunningham 'Tank Treatment," Journal of The American Medical Association, Vol. 90 No. i8, May 5, 1928. Reprinted by permission of Journal of The American Medical Association.

Hyperbaric Oxygenation—Potentials and Problems (1963). Reprinted by permission of the publisher, The National Academy of Sciences.

The Hyperbaric Medicine Newsletter, Vols. I-VIII, ed. Dr. Harry J. Alvis. Reprinted by permission of the editor.

"Clinical Hyperbaric Oxygenation with Severe Oxygen Toxicity," Drs. Robert L. Funson, Herbert A. Saltzman, Wirt W. Smith, Robert E. Whalen, Suydam Osterhout, and Roy T. Parker, The New England Journal of Medicine, Vol. 273 No. 8, Aug. 19, 1965. Reprinted by permission of The New England Journal of Medicine and the authors.

Directory of World-Wide, Shore-based Hyperbaric Chambers, Vols. I and II, January 1971. Reprinted by permission of Supervisor of Diving, United States Navy.

ISBN: 979-822-45219-51
LIBRARY OF CONGRESS CATALOG CARD NUMBER
73-79721

ACKNOWLEDGEMENTS

I wish to express my gratitude to the many individuals and organizations who freely gave information, and especially to Dr Harry J. Alvis of Buffalo, New York, and Dr. Cornelia M. Dettmer of Cincinnati, both of whom not only served as medical consultants but also reviewed the manuscript for technical accuracy, though neither should bear any responsibility for the author's interpretations or conclusions.

For their substantial research contributions my sincere thanks to Dr. George B. Hart and Mrs. Alice Gaul, of Long Beach, California; to Dr. Eric P. Kindwall, Dr. Carl Zenz, and Dr. Edgar End, of Milwaukee; to Dr. Louis R. M. Del Guercio, Anthony Scala, Dr. Dennis R. Filippone, George S. Beakley, Bob Cornish, Mrs. Constance Warshoff, and Dr. James A. Hogan, of Livingston, New Jersey; to Dr. Julius H. Jacobson II, Dr. Howard A. Rusk, Dr. Theobald Reich, Leonard Diller, Ph.D., Myron Youdin, Miss Nancy Tuckerman, secretary to Jacqueline Kennedy Onassis, C. G. Coburn, program director of the John A. Hartford Foundation, of New York; to Dr. Jack Van Elk, Dr. Luke R. Pascale, Dr. Morris Fishbein, of Chicago; to Frank Chappell and Oliver Field of the American Medical Association; and to John T. Mahoney of the Vacudyne Corp., of Chicago.

To Wesley Peoples, Arthur Smith, and James Price, of Bethlehem, Pennsylvania; to Major William F. Long, of Dallas; to Dr. William F. Bernhard, Dr. James E. Drorbaugh, Jim Carr, Ross A. McFarland, Ph.D., William Keith, Ph.D., Herbert Shaw, Richard Wolfe of Harvard's Countway Library, William J. Brennan of Children's Medical Center, of Boston; to Dr. Alan P. Thal and Miss Helen Sims of Kansas City, Kansas; to Dr. Ralph Hall, Miss Merre Shane and Mrs. Charles Dennie, of Kansas City, Missouri; and to Dr. R. Adams Cowley and Jerome Touhy, of Baltimore, Maryland.

To Dr. Claude Hitchcock of Minneapolis, Minnesota; to Dr. John H. Turgeson of Madison, Wisconsin; to Dr. Herbert Saltzman and Joe Sigler of Duke University, of Durham, North Carolina; to Cliff Marr of Battelle Memorial Institute and Dr. Charles Billings, of Columbus, Ohio: to Dr. Albert R. Behnke of San Francisco; to Eleanor Jacobs, Ph.D., Dr. Edward H. Lanphier, of Buffalo, New York; to Dr. Sreedhar Nair and Richard Imbruce, Ph.D., of Norwalk, Connecticut; to Ruth Epstein of Cincinnati General Hospital Library, Dr. Saul Benison of the University of Cincinnati, James Blair, Jr, Mrs. Richard Kreuter, Dr. Eldridge Baker, of Cincinnati; to John Y. Brown, Sr., of Lexington and Louisville, Kentucky.

Also, to Senator Harrison Williams of New Jersey, Andy Rothman, LeRoy Goldman, Bill Oriole, Mrs. Everett M. Dirksen, Lynda L. Cahoon, John A. Blake, Ph.D., of the National Library of Medicine, Captain Ben Hastings, U. S. Navy, and Dr. Henry Gannon, of Washington, D.C.

My appreciation, too, for the helping hands lent by colleagues in the press: Mildred Whiteaker of the San Antonio (Texas) News-Express; Cruise Palmer of the Kansas City (Missouri) Star; Arville Schaleben of the Milwaukee Journal; Richard Hollander of the Scripps-Howard Washington Bureau; Creed Black of the Philadelphia Inquirer; Tom Boardman and Bob Yonkers of The Cleveland (Ohio) Press; Joan Rice of the Akron (Ohio) Beacon-Journal; Julius Frandsen of United Press International, Washington, D.C.; Don Weaver of Worthington, Ohio; and Carl West, Randy Cochran, and Nancy Taylor of The Kentucky Post staff.

The family of Dr. Orval J. Cunningham was gracious and generous with their time and historic memorabilia, for which I warmly thank his son Orval, Jr., of Natick, Massachusetts, daughter Dorothy (Mrs. Leslie N. II) Duryea, and widow Grace, both of Fullerton, California. Valuable help on this portion of the book was given by their friend H. J. Rand III, of Cleveland, Ohio.

My gratitude also for the assistance of my wife, Elzene; daughter, Carol Ann Weisenfeld, of Miami, Florida, and sister-in-law, Edwina Cline, of Houston, Texas. I am indebted to my editor, Diane Cleaver, for her patient and expert guidance.

For C. A. Dwyer, Jr., M.D.
...mantener los viejos amigos

INTRODUCTION

THE UNCERTAIN MIRACLE
By
Vance Trimble

Republished in 2023

By

I.P. Semmelweis Memorial Publications
LLC

PREFACE

This is a book that has needed writing for a long time. Vance Trimble has not found this an easy nor simple matter. The required research has taken him into all manner of byways including locating elderly relatives and friends of certain individuals. Beyond this he has had to educate himself in the ways and mannerisms of the medical profession, first of all overcoming their built-in predisposition of negativism toward the reportorial craft. But Trimble is more than a craftsman. He was able to bring his reportorial skills, which are great, along with his unusual degree of humaneness into this scene.

As a practitioner and believer in this form of treatment I know he has dealt well with the essential facts. While this may not be the complete source book for historians, there can be no doubt the author has brought light to some murky corners of the background. His research files would be a compilation almost any medical library would be pleased to add to their collection. Above all he has brought a readable exposition to a much misunderstood area of current medical practice. Hyperbaric medicine is no "fountain of youth" nor "raising from the grave" exercise but there is a genuine role for this modality and Vance Trimble has contributed a highly interesting, pleasantly readable account of what the field can do and how it is done. My personal thanks go to Vance Trimble for having persisted in completing this formidable and needed document.

Harry J. Alvis, M.D.
    Submarine Medical Officer, USN
    Associate Clinical Professor,
    School of Medicine,
    State University of New York at Buffalo

Consultant, Hyperbaric Medicine Veterans' Administration
Hospital Buffalo, New York
Millard Fillmore Hospital
Buffalo, New York

Foreword

I stand on the shoulders of giants! Pity the hapless souls who have not endlessly regaled themselves as children, immersed in hero worship of the great luminaries of yesteryear, the intellectual pillars of thought, of literature, of deed, the pioneers of science.

There are many names that we keep on the tip of the tongue, that writers carry on the lead of their pencil—Hippocrates, Darwin, Einstein, Pasteur. But what of the legions of unsung heroes—Manfred von Ardenne, Jean-Baptiste Lamarck, Claude Bernard, Otto Warburg?

Indeed, Dr. Orval J. Cunningham was assuredly one of those unsung heroes.

Who amongst us has delved deeply into the works, into the minds, of these legends? In "The Uncertain Miracle," published in 1974 by Vance Trimble, who won the Pulitzer Prize in 1960 for investigative journalism, republished in 2023 by the International Hyperbaric Medical Foundation through the I.P. Semmelweis Memorial Publications, LLC, we take a deep dive (all puns intended) not only into the thoughts and work of Dr Cunningham, but also reveal a brief taste of the insufferable trials and tribulations he was subjected to as penalties for challenging medical orthodoxy.

Not because he was wrong, mind you, rather because he rescued people from needless suffering and terminal diseases using hyperbarics instead of pharmaceuticals. Reflecting his own personal experiences, Albert Einstein quipped, *"Great spirits have always encountered violent opposition from mediocre minds. The mediocre mind is incapable of understanding the man who refuses to bow blindly to conventional prejudices and chooses instead to express his opinions courageously and honestly."*

As a research scientist, my original antiaging, tissue and organ regeneration R&D over the past 51 years was built on a foundation of solid bedrock proffered by the original works of all the great minds captioned above, along with many more not listed. Condensation, amalgamation, contemplation, and integration of such a smorgasbord of originality breeds more original thought. We must not deceive ourselves. We must not allow suppression and censorship in any nuance nor context. We must not succumb to hubris. Science has barely scratched the surface of the way the universe works, of human health. All we must do is listen and pay close attention, to think deeply, and not be distracted by the extraneous noise and chatter of contemporary society. I have been richly blessed to be allowed to stand on the shoulders of giants! The possibilities remain limitless!

Humbly,

International Hyperbaric Medical Foundation

Dr Merrel Holley, DSc, President

&

The Tissue & Organ Regeneration Institute (a 501(c)3)

Antiaging, Tissue & Organ Regeneration

Dr Merrel Holley, DSc, Senior Research Scientist

Medical Advice Disclaimer

DISCLAIMER: THE IHMF DOES NOT PROVIDE MEDICAL ADVICE

The information, including but not limited to, text, graphics, images and other material contained on this website, publications and responses to questions are for informational purposes only, typically citing published research papers. No material provided from the IHMF or its agents is intended to be a substitute for professional medical advice, diagnosis or treatment. Always seek the advice of your physician or other qualified healthcare provider with any questions you may have regarding a medical condition or treatment and before undertaking a new healthcare regimen, and never disregard professional medical advice or delay in seeking it because of something you have read on this website or responses to questions.

Forward

I entered the universe of hyperbaric science the way most people do: watching the movies and adventures of Jaques Cousteau, oceanaut, on Sunday nights. For a young boy raised in poverty by a single mom east of Los Angeles, CA, it was a glorious escape from life's difficulties.

Years later, in college on the opposite coast, it was a natural progression to get trained and certified to dive off the coast of Gloucester, MA. My recreational diving became the nemesis for any tasty lobster I could find. Scuba diving in real life turned out to be a thousand percent better than anything books or television could only hint at. The overwhelming sense of well-being, adventure and the required focus and skill probably developed me more as a young man than all my other experiences combined.

Many years later my mother was diagnosed with Parkinson's Disease.

Thus began a highly emotional and desperate quest to help her. I quickly discovered the *allowable* medical approach to Parkinson's was pretty much limited to a handful of expensive pills. The prognosis would always be her body adapting to the medication and the progression of the disease continuing. After exhausting every known medical approach to helping her and not being satisfied with the "go home and slowly die shaking" or "be a medicated zombie at the taxpayers' expense" statements, I pursued HBOT, or Hyperbaric Oxygen Therapy.

Not surprisingly, HBOT for Parkinson's Disease was denied by both doctors and insurance companies. Not that it couldn't help, it was simply not on their allowable schedule. It took me many hours of frustrating conversations to understand that most doctors have been transitioned into providers, and providers only provide based on permission from a strange conglomeration of the American Medical

Association, insurance companies, the Trial Lawyers Association of America, Big Pharma and to a secondary extent, directed academics at leading universities.

I had pursued HBOT, not because of any study or recommendation, but because it was the closest thing to my diving experience where anytime I got below thirty feet in saltwater, I always felt wonderful. I felt great and had a mild euphoria for a day afterwards. I am a simple man in many ways. For me, if my body feels good, it is good. My mother felt terrible all the time, her muscles ached constantly from non-stop tremors, her sleep was short and wretched, she was fighting depression, she couldn't start and stop well, her balance was bad, and life was getting difficult. Medication merely masked her symptoms by giving her others. I would do anything to help her feel better.

With the help of some wonderfully skilled friends over the course of a year I built a multi-place Hyperbaric Atmosphere Chamber. If I were to write about the process, expense, regulations, certifications etc., it would take an entire book. It is close to impossible for an individual to both safely and legally do it. However, my day job at the time was pastoring a church and I knew how to pray. I also had an advantage that most people don't: my friends build submarines, run nuclear power plants, build oil platforms, and I was surrounded with engineers and retiring scientists. One of my friends, Norman an inventor and accomplished welder, simply believed in what I was trying to accomplish and devoted himself to the immense project. It wouldn't have happened without him.

The first session of dry diving my mother to fifty-two feet for forty minutes at depth removed her muscle pain. The second dive ended her shaking for quite some time. By the fifth dive she walked better. In under ten dives I gave her back her car keys and she could use the stairs, get up and down from the floor with her grandkids, and teach Sunday School again.

My mother went ninety-percent symptom free for seven years, with no medication. She got her life back. If she did three sessions a week, her disease did not progress. Five sessions per week showed reversal. To my extreme frustration, Hyperbaric Atmosphere Saturation (what I do) does not cure Parkinsons. But her doctor told me that he believed my system was the greatest palliative care in the United States for PD.

Today I have ten staff members and multiple volunteers and my company, Hyperbaric Fitness of Swanzey, NH is averaging twenty-five to forty clients per day for dry diving. Non-Medical, Health and Wellness is our focus. The stem cell increase coupled with immune system support, breathing aid and detoxification that occurs in Hyperbaric Atmosphere has been a real-life health hack for our clients for eleven years.

This book is of inestimable value. I read it for the first time in 2022, eleven years after I started my journey. I would be much further ahead by now if I had this knowledge. I very much identify with the early pioneers and doctors in this book as to the challenges they faced. Divers, doctors, researchers and inventors should all read this book for their knowledge base. The public should read it for its inspiration.

Warning: It will take you into the universe of possibilities and your life may never be the same.

Joseph Mabe, Owner

Hyperbaric Fitness, LLC of Swanzey, NH

1

WHEN IT'S LIFE OR DEATH

On a sunny afternoon in late March 1968, Dr. George B. Hart hurried along a second-floor corridor in the U. S. Naval Hospital in Long Beach, California. At precisely four by his watch, he turned into the south-wing assembly hall, his jaw out-thrust. Twenty or thirty others milled about finding seats for the Conference on Combat Casualties. Those who observed Hart's entry understood the frustration reflected in his scowl, for the whole medical staff shared it.

They were grappling with a very tough case—the tall Marine corporal who had sunken, pleading eyes, a gaunt pain-wracked face, and a frail, rotting body. He was young, and should be getting well, but the doctors weren't doing him any good. He was practically a living skeleton. His prospects were poor; the corporal was, in fact, dying.

Hart brusquely rapped the blackboard with a piece of chalk. As Chief of Surgery, this meeting was his show. He had initiated these monthly conferences the previous fall, with discussion limited to truly complicated cases coming in from the Vietnam battlefields. Hart was trying to achieve two goals: first, to find some better course of treatment for any war wounded not doing well under conventional therapy; and secondly, in that way to further the training of reservist physicians assigned to him.

Most of the doctors assembled before George Babe Hart were quite young. Only thirty-eight years old himself, he felt almost a graybeard in this company. From the University of Texas Medical School, he had gone directly into the Navy as a physician in 1956. Already he had served as Chief of Surgery at two other Navy installations, now held the rank of full commander and would advance by 1972 to captain.

Waiting for the doctors to settle down, Hart looked them over admiringly, impressed by the enormous storehouse of hard-earned medical knowledge collectively reposing in these minds. Yet their combined skill, he reflected ruefully, was doing precious damn little for Corporal James Joseph Helfer.

On his way to the assembly, Hart had looked in again on Helfer. In the six months since the corporal had been brought to Long Beach, Hart had seen him at least fifty times. Though gravely wounded, Helfer had arrived weighing about 160 pounds. Now he was a bony, shrunken human shell, barely 80 pounds!

At a signal from Hart, the orthopedist strode to the front and began slipping the patient's latest X-ray films under the viewing screen clips. The Chief of Surgery sat down to watch and listen grimly, hopeful the upcoming discussion might somehow spawn a fresh clue for solving their baffling problem.

The orthopedic surgeon recited Helfer's case history, Navy medical SOP, but practically everyone present already knew the full story. It had been reviewed at each previous Combat Casualty Conference, the most discussed case, the most stubborn, the most disappointing. For a dozen other complicated casualties, successful new treatments were devised; but this one defied the doctors' finest efforts.

Helfer's chart gave all the basics: age, twenty-two; height, six feet two; hometown, Covina, California. Wounded July 15, 1967, during skirmish in the mountains north of Khe Sanh. He was the gunner in a US Marine tank guarding the vital road to Hill 881 where an American radar outpost kept watch across the border into North Vietnam. Helfer climbed out of his tank, and instantly was hit in the lower back by an enemy rocket.

A buddy dragged him to cover, and a medic put compress bandages over gaping holes where the four-inch shell had gone through his body and called in a rescue helicopter. He was evacuated to Da Nang, where surgeons found extensive damage. His intestines were mangled, one kidney ruptured, multiple nerves severed or bruised, and his spine above the pelvis had been viciously scraped by the projectile.

The military doctors feared the rocket's concussion might have done additional damage they couldn't then detect; but they patched him up fairly well, performing a colostomy because of the bowel trauma. He was sent aboard the hospital ship U.S.S. Sanctuary for a few weeks, then flown back to the United States, and admitted on September 16, 1967, to Long Beach Naval Hospital. Helfer had arrived in critical condition and, despite all the doctors could do, went steadily downhill. His primary wounds, fortunately, had generally healed. But the enemy rocket's assault on his backbone had brought on the present life-threatening complication. This was chronic osteomyelitis, a terrible disease that causes bone to literally rot and exude a putrid ooze through an open wound known as a sinus. Helfer's lower spine was affected, specifically the fourth and fifth lumbar vertebrae and the sacrum. He had a large decubitus ulcer, a bedsore.

The Long Beach doctors began vigorous treatment at once. The orthopedist inserted a catheter into the sinus and irrigated the infected bones with antibiotic solutions. That had little effect. Helfer was given more antibiotics, steroids, hormones. He required one blood transfusion a week.

A special diet was prescribed to try to build up his weight, but he ran a fever and his condition continued to deteriorate. At the first Combat Casualty Conference, it was decided to try a sequestrectomy surgery to remove pockets of dead bone from the diseased area. This operation was performed not only once, but thrice.

Nothing the Navy doctors tried made any headway against the disease. But they didn't give up. The orthopedist called his old professor at UCLA for advice and consulted other medical notables around the country. The neurosurgeon also sought outside counsel. Neither got any beneficial suggestions.

While this March conference was in progress, over in the north wing, Helfer lay flat on his back, suffering great pain, partially paralyzed, down to half his normal weight, and seized by a frightening new complication, a critical spinal inflammation called ascending myelitis. Soon, crippling nerve paralysis would endanger his vital organs.

When the doctors concluded their discussion and filed out of the assembly hall, the Helfer case was still strictly status quo. Nobody had come up with a new slant on treatment.

"It was plain as the nose on your face." Hart recalled later. "Corporal Helfer was going down the tubes. He was dying—and we didn't know how to save him."

Hart felt sympathy for the orthopedist and the neurosurgeon. They were young but good and they had tried their best. After all, chronic osteomyelitis had always been a difficult disease; he didn't recall that any physician had ever had much luck arresting it.

Hart pondered the dilemma as he walked to his office. There surely must be some way to save Helfer. Abruptly he decided to assume personal responsibility for the case.

Next morning, he instructed the hospital librarian to comb the medical literature on chronic osteomyelitis—everything published anywhere in the world. A few days later extracts from medical journals started flowing across his desk. He scanned four or five articles a day. This went on about three weeks, but nothing he read looked helpful. Meanwhile Corporal Helfer got sicker.

In mid-April, when Hart had almost abandoned hope, the library sent him a paper delivered at the Third International Conference on Hyperbaric Medicine in the fall of 1965 at Duke University, Durham, North Carolina.

Dr. David J. D. Perrins of London had reported to the conference that he and four other British surgeons had treated chronic osteomyelitis with hyperbaric oxygenation and the results were fantastically favorable. The British doctors reported a 75 per cent cure rate. Hart was dumbfounded. Why hadn't he heard about something this sensational? He'd been in medicine twelve years; he'd done several thousand surgical procedures; and yet at this moment he felt as backward as a freshman med student. It was embarrassing to be so unaware of hyperbaric oxygenation—especially if it offered new hope in this complicated case.

Hart knew little about hyperbaric medicine. He could recall no mention of it during medical school or his internship in Boston, nor during his two years at Camp Lejeune, North Carolina. He spent a four years' residency in general surgery at Portsmouth, New Hampshire, General Hospital, and there he had read some articles about hyperbaric oxygenation, which is generally abbreviated as HBO in the medical journals but was not impressed.

Neither was he impressed at St. Albans Naval Hospital Island, New York, where a staff doctor used a small pressure chamber to experiment with diseased rats. While he was finishing his thoracic surgery residency at St. Albans, Hart had read about a doctor in Amsterdam performing surgery in a hyperbaric chamber, an air-tight vessel similar to the decompression tanks (also referred to as recompression tanks) that have been in use for more than 100 years to pressurize deep-sea divers and cure them of the "bends". Doctors at St. Albans discussed over coffee the Dutch surgeon's achievement, but Hart idly shrugged it off as a technique that seemed of little real use in his field of medicine.

Now on closer look, hyperbaric medicine made clear sense. Hart had resisted Navy efforts to lure him into submarine and diving medicine, although he was a scuba diver. He had taken up the sport in the Gulf of Mexico during medical school days at Galveston, Texas. Scuba diving had familiarized him with decompression tanks and given him practical experience in how human physiology reacts to pressurization. He had observed treatment of sick divers in decompression tanks in which the atmospheric pressure would be pumped up two or three times greater than sea level normal. Under such pressure, the diver would instantly and dramatically increase the oxygen content of his blood by inhaling pure oxygen through a face mask. The pressure acts on gas molecules to literally compress more oxygen into the diver's blood stream.

Hart could visualize hyperbaric oxygenation benefiting someone like Helfer in two ways. First, any oxygen-starved cell in his body, particularly in the brain, would be revived and function better. Secondly, osteomyelitis usually is caused by anaerobic bacteria which can exist only where there is little or no oxygen. Thus, obviously use of the hyperbaric oxygen treatment should knock out the microbes that were destroying the corporal's lower spine. Hart remembered the Amsterdam surgeon referred to this treatment as "drenching" the body with oxygen.

Up to this point in his career, Hart had never thought it all of exploring the technique of "drenching" with oxygen. Previous HBO articles had left him uncertain and decidedly negative. His reaction to the article he now read was entirely different. It had real substance and was authored by five British surgeons who had delivered it before a prestigious international conclave.

To a surgeon agonizing over his frustrating inability to rescue a Vietnam casualty from the jaws of death, the British results looked sensational. Dr. Perrins and his colleagues had treated twenty-four cases of chronic osteomyelitis, each of which had a discharging sinus as did Corporal Helfer. Seventeen of these patients healed totally, four were substantially helped, and only three were apparently uninfluenced by the treatment.

As Hart read through the case histories, he felt a surge of hope for the dying corporal. One British patient, seventy years old, had suffered forty years from a large draining sinus on his hip that made him a cripple. After intermittent treatments in the pressure tank totaling forty-nine hours, he walked unassisted, and the wound began closing. Only fourteen hours in the chamber cured a fifty-three-year-old man who for twenty years had chronic osteomyelitis of the upper end of the left tibia.

Dr. Perrins and his colleagues wrote:

Based on our limited experience to date we have the impression that hyperbaric oxygenation can favorably influence the course of a persistent sinus in chronic osteomyelitis, and that given sufficient exposure most but not all cases will heal, at least temporarily. Present evidence does not justify an assumption, however, that the effects on the sinus necessarily represent an influence on the underlying disease process. We do not know whether the beneficial effects we have observed were achieved by (1) influencing the oxygenation of the infected area, (2) inhibiting the growth of the organisms, (3) potentiating the action of the antibiotics, or (4) an interrelation of these factors.

It wasn't known why oxygen "drenching" was causing the osteomyelitis to heal but the tank treatment was working better than 75 per cent of the time. Hart thought about the current odds his medical staff was giving Helfer for survival—maybe one chance in ten thousand. Now things could be different, the British odds on getting a cure were three to one. All Hart needed to do was to get the corporal into an oxygen chamber.

Long Beach Naval Hospital is just off the freeway in a suburb of Los Angeles, about twenty miles from the waterfront. It had nothing remotely resembling a hyperbaric chamber. Hart felt certain that the Terminal Island Navy Yard in Long Beach harbor would have a decompression tank for use by its divers. Essentially that would be the same as a hyperbaric chamber.

Hart lifted the phone to dial the Navy Yard, suddenly paused. Frowning, he replaced the receiver. He just remembered one section of Navy regs—a Navy hospital can't treat anyone with any unproven drug or procedure without prior approval from the Navy Bureau in Washington. What about hyperbaric oxygenation? Was it an experimental treatment, or a proven drug? Hart considered Helfer's rapid deterioration and weighed that against the time it would take to wade through all the red tape between Long Beach and Washington, and back. Hart shrugged, and again picked up the phone.

He asked for the Navy Yard's submarine and diving medical officer. Lieutenant Commander Frank Depenbusch came on the line. Yes, there was a standard decompression chamber on Terminal Island. Hart said he would be right over. At the Navy Yard he explained Helfer's plight to Depenbusch and showed him the British medical report. Depenbusch readily agreed it would be a good idea to treat Helfer in the decompression tank—but mentioned a couple of hitches. Nobody could use a Navy tank without passing a diver's physical exam; and also, somebody had to pay the tank's two tenders, Civil Service employees, twenty-five dollars an hour each. Those were Navy regs. It was unthinkable that Helfer could pass any kind of physical; but Depenbusch suggested a way around that. The shipyard's C.O. had authority to circumvent the regulations. Hart looked up the C.O.—Captain C. Monroe Hart (no relation)—and won him over. Then he did what he calls a "fast-talking con job" on the two tenders.

To Helfer, the prospect of a hopeful new treatment brought no great joy. He was too weak, too feverish, and too dispirited to react one way or the other. It took a week to set everything up, Hart fretting all the while about Helfer's increasing frailty. Hart began to doubt that the corporal would be strong enough to stand the pressure; some very ill patients cannot. They'd just have to see.

On the morning of April 22, 1968, an ambulance delivered Helfer, with Hart riding at his side, to the Navy Yard. The decompression chamber was an unprepossessing black iron tank resembling a boiler, six and a half feet in diameter and sixteen and a half feet long. Two tenders had to stoop to carry Helfer on his stretcher through the entry hatch at one end. Depenbusch followed, clanged shut the door, dogged it, and set the valves to let the pressure build up to twice seal-level atmosphere, which is equivalent to the water weight a diver feels at a depth of thirty-three feet.

Through a glass porthole, Hart looked in to watch Depenbusch instruct the corporal how to execute the Valsalva maneuver. This required Helfer to pinch his nostrils and swallow to clear his Eustachian tubes, thus preventing the build-up of painful pressure against the eardrums.

Depenbusch took down an oronasal mask connected to the wall by flexible tubing and adjusted it against Helfer's face so he could breathe piped-in pure oxygen during his two-hour "dive"—as time spent inside the chamber under pressure is called. Hart and Depenbusch had decided to adhere to the time and pressure schedule Dr. Perrins had used successfully.

Everything seemed to be starting out okay, but Hart watched the control board's big clock anxiously, and frequently peered through the porthole. Inside Helfer lay relaxed, the oxygen mask snug to his face. Hart sat down, and kept his fingers crossed. Finally, he heard the pop of a valve somewhere back of the tank and the hiss of escaping air. Two hours had gone by, and a few minutes later, the tenders carried Helfer out. Hart moved up for a close look. Helfer seemed better; his skin looked pinker and fresher than it had for a long time.

He had tolerated the pressure well and would be able to take the pressure dives every day. The second and third treatments seemed to give Helfer a little spirit, and when he emerged from the fourth dive, his brown eyes were alert, he lifted his head and smiled weakly.

Hart wanted to whoop for joy. Now there was no doubt about it—the tank was whipping the bugs. But it took many more weeks of dives and therapy before Helfer finally overcame the disease. First, his fever vanished, then he started making his own blood again, and his decubitus ulcer healed. Drainage from his osteomyelitis fistula began to diminish, he gained weight, and finally he was up and on his feet. After thirty-eight dives, the osteomyelitis drainage had ceased altogether, and the once terrible wound was healed. Helfer was well enough to be discharged from this hospital.

The medical staff was elated. The orthopedist promptly suggested the same tank treatments for other Long Beach Navy Hospital patients suffering from chronic osteomyelitis. One had acquired the infection in 1939 after a mine accident and the other, a chaplain, had hobbled around two years because his infected leg wouldn't heal. Hart sent both to the tank and they too got well.

The irony of all this disturbed Hart. He kept wondering why he had been unaware of the tank treatment. Was it merely a personal shortcoming, or could it be that many other doctors were in the dark and would have to blindly grope for the same dim path and discover hyperbaric medicine literally via the back door? Suspecting as much, he inquired around and sadly concluded that probably seven of ten physicians in general practice were just as unaware of HBO as he had been.

Such a situation struck Hart as inexcusable; further reading of medical journals told him that HBO had been rather extensively used in some cities in the United States since the early 1960s, and, to a limited degree, even since 1918. Not only that, but it had also been reported effective against twenty or so disease and trauma conditions. And yet, even in the late 1960s, the vast majority of America's 300,000 physicians and surgeons seemed unimpressed or uninformed—or, tragically, both.

Convinced he had tardily discovered the most neglected and underrated tool in the armamentarium of modern medicine, Hart set about become one of the country's most tireless HBO researchers and evangelists. First, he needed to square accounts with his Navy superiors. He reported his stunning results to the hospital C.O., confessed to short-circuiting red tape, and asked approval to continue using tank treatments. The pleased hospital commandant congratulated Hart, dispatched the request to Washington, and drew $2,000 from his fund to reimburse the tenders who were running the tank.

Navy Bureau admirals were unhappy about not being consulted. They stirred up quite a storm. It didn't faze Hart. By the time Washington finally granted formal approval, Hart had already treated sixty more cases.

Long Beach Navy Hospital's belated discovery of high-pressure oxygen's great healing power is, unfortunately, rather typical. The curious history of hyperbaric medicine is dappled by murky shadows of scientific foot-dragging, violent skepticism, long barren stretches of total neglect. And the tragic consequence is that today's apathy and hesitation exacts a cruel toll. Every year, thousands who could be saved by tank treatments die needlessly. Some authorities privately put the estimate as high as ten thousand.

Why then is hyperbaric therapy so ignored? Is modern medicine too conservative, unwilling to accept change? Too busy? Too blasé and sophisticated? Too skeptical? There are no easy answers, but a little light can be shed on the underlying problems by examining the experiences of a few other physicians in the field.

Milwaukee offers a class illustration of harmful skepticism. Luckily, Milwaukee is today a leading HBO center, with three active chambers. The city easily could have acquired that distinction forty years ago—if its doctors had been less dubious.

Their golden opportunity came in 1927 when excavation began for Milwaukee's huge new sewer system. The city fronts Lake Michigan presenting the constant threat of the lake undermining and flooding the fresh-dug tunnels. To prevent this, the shafts were filled with compressed air; the "sandhogs" went down through air locks to dig in pressurized holes seventy-five feet beneath the streets.

It was risky work. When such a caisson system was first used in this country in 1878 to tunnel under the Hudson River at New York City, many diggers fell ill. In Milwaukee, too, some diggers unexpectedly keeled over after coming to the surface. Joseph Sebalz, fifty-five years old, left the night shift in the tunnel on March 24, 1927, and collapsed while going home on the streetcar. They rushed him to the hospital and diagnosed the problem; he had decompression sickness, the "bends." Sebalz died, and so did several more of the sewer excavators.

Physicians at that time knew little about this strange malady. The cause, at least, had been isolated: nitrogen bubbles which did not dissipate normally and became trapped in blood or tissues of caisson workers or divers who emerged too rapidly from being under pressure. To avoid the bends, sandhogs were required to emerge from their pressurized tunnels via an air lock. In this they emerge from their pressurized tunnels via an air lock. In this they rested in fifteen-to-thirty-minute stages while air pressure was gradually reduced until it equaled the normal outside atmosphere. These formulas were inexact, and doctors did not exchange data on a sickness affecting such a limited worker class.

But this situation became so alarming in 1928 that health officials in Milwaukee ordered a decompression chamber built. The only known effective way to treat the bends was to recompress the ailing sandhog and start over on the gradual stages of decompression to allow time for the trapped nitrogen to dissipate normally through his lungs.

Milwaukee authorities decided the city needed its own decompression chamber and gave a boilermaker $5000 to make a seven by eighteen-foot chamber. But the Depression intervened, the tunnel work dragged, and the tank was not ready until 1931. Even then, it wasn't used but sat idle in the basement of Milwaukee County Emergency Hospital until 1936. Dr. Edgar End, twenty-six, stumbled upon the tank, used only for storage of junk tables. End, amateur diver during Marquette University student days, saw the iron monster as a tool for research. He promptly got it going, just as the sewer work resumed, and Milwaukee sandhogs, no longer died of the bends. End has kept the chamber going ever since nearly forty years.

And when he wasn't curing sewer workers, End turned the tank into an experimental laboratory. He devised sophisticated oxygen-helium mixes for deep-sea divers, explored high pressure physiology, sometimes using himself as a human guinea pig. Quite early, he discovered his simple tank could tremendously elevate oxygen content of the blood. He tried to tell other doctors. Few would listen.

End read medical journal accounts of compressed-air therapy in two or three other cities, but nothing seemed to be conclusive. So, he kept experimenting in his tank with mice, rabbits, and dogs. He made a sensational discovery about carbon monoxide. Inside the tank, this poison could be washed out of a victim's blood ten to twenty-five times faster than the conventional method—which was to administer oxygen by face mask, of course, at sea-level pressure. End and Dr. Chester W. Long tested the new process on animals for two years. Then they unveiled their treatment at County Emergency Hospital's annual staff meeting on February 5, 1942. Nobody seemed to buy the idea. End also proposed his new therapy in the

American Journal of Industrial Medicine. That article likewise drew a ho-hum response.

Milwaukee foolishly ignored this new treatment for nearly two decades, as did virtually every American doctor. Then during the 1960s HBO upsurge in Europe, their identical treatment was rediscovered by doctors at Western Infirmary in Glasgow, Scotland. Belatedly impressed, Milwaukee now has the finest carbon-monoxide rescue system in the nation, utilizing two large modern hyperbaric chambers across town at St. Luke's Hospital run by Dr. Eric P. Kindwall, incidentally once a teen-age protégé of End's.

None of those early rebuffs seemed to daunt End. He kept studying oxygen and experimenting with pressure. It became clear to him that breathing 100 per cent oxygen under double or triple atmospheric pressure would help patients with ischemia, oxygen-starved tissue, or with impaired blood circulation. He was one of the first investigators to recognize the value of tank treatments for gangrene. Likewise, he saw that HBO would enrich the vascular bed under risky skin grafts and thus lessen the danger that these transplants might not "take." So, when the son of a Milwaukee surgeon crashed through a glass door and suffered horrible gashes, End volunteered help. A large flap of torn skin hung on the lad's face by only a thin pedicle. This fragile strip of flesh provided the only link to the boy's blood circulation that could keep the skin patch alive until new arteries developed. And the pedicle appeared to be dying. End suggested pressurizing the boy in his tank to escalate the healing. The distraught father agreed, and in a few dives the skin flap took nicely.

The surgeon was so impressed he came to End a few weeks later about a patient, a woman teacher, fifty-four, suffering diabetic gangrene of the lower extremities, an infection brought on by closure of peripheral small blood vessels. To halt the gangrene's spread, the surgeon had amputated her left leg at mid-thigh. Now the disease was attacking her right leg. Her foot was black, the rotting instep had burst open, and dark splotches climbed toward her knee.

Could the tank do anything for her? End thought it could, at the least the oxygen-enrichment of her blood would reveal a clear line of demarcation between the part of the leg that was necrotic, actually dead, and live tissue. End suggested that such a development might permit a low amputation, perhaps only of her foot.

After only two dives the teacher's leg turned pink; her foot, too, lightened. The surgeon conceded that the tank had done its work well and took his patient away. Two weeks later End chanced to meet the surgeon. "How much did you amputate?" End asked.

"None! Ed, that woman has already gone home. I didn't amputate at all. Just trimmed a little necrotic tissue off her instep. Her leg and foot cleared up completely. That old boiler of yours whipped the gangrene."

Convincing evidence? Apparently not to that particular surgeon, End later lamented. For some reason, he never sent other patients to the tank.

Operating with his little bargain-basement tank virtually in the shadow of large gleaming chambers price-tagged at $300,000, End continues active in hyperbaric medicine, is saving lives with his simple "boiler" and still probing the intriguing mysteries of high-pressure physiology. He has, unfortunately, tended to be too far ahead of his time. When he discovered HBO's amazing effectiveness in the treatment of strokes and senility, End wrote an article in 1967 to submit to the Journal of the American Medical Association. It was rejected as "too absurd" for publication. The JAMA editors who turned it down may be now a trifle red-faced. Leading experts today verify End's findings and believe HBO well may turn out to be medicine's hottest weapon in the important battle against the stroke and senility syndromes.

The history of hyperbaric medicine in Kansas City is even more ludicrous. America's first major clinical use of pressurized oxygenation began there in 1918. Dr. Orval J. Cunningham built a crude tank to treat World War I flu epidemic victims. He cured some patients, and later experimented so successfully on other diseases that he reigned for nearly twenty years as the nation's most intensive, and controversial hyperbarist.

Yet until 1969, no Kansas City hospital had ever installed hyperbaric equipment. In that year, a cardiologist from Kansas City's St. Luke's Hospital, Dr. James Crockett, went abroad. In Holland, he saw one-patient Vickers chambers used in heart-attack cases. He was so impressed, he came home and persuaded St. Luke's, which was 634 beds in Kansas City's largest hospital, to buy two of the British-built chambers.

Doctors at St. Luke's have used their two tanks effectively against gas gangrene, carbon monoxide poisoning, sickle-cell crisis, myocardial infarction (heart attacks), and to promote the heading of skin grafts. However, the chairman of the hospital's hyperbaric department, Dr. Ralph Hall, says that staff doctors nonetheless view their results "with a healthy skepticism."

A recent near tragedy in Cincinnati points up the alarming degree of ignorance about HBO prevalent today even among well-intentioned physicians who gladly would call on the tank's magic if only they knew about it.

Twin girls were born by Caesarean section on June 14, 1972, at Cincinnati's Good Samaritan Hospital to Mrs. Richard Kreuter. Her first babies were fine and healthy. Her obstetrician, Dr. Eldridge Baker, considered it a fairly routine delivery. For a couple of days Mrs. Kreuter, small, pretty, and only twenty-four years old, was making what doctors' term "an uneventful recovery."

Suddenly she developed a fever. Checking for the cause, Baker removed the bandage from her abdomen and got a severe shock.

Both edges of her incision had turned black. He couldn't account for this unexpected complication, but he feared some infection causing gangrene had developed. He sent a smear and culture from the black wound to the laboratory and without waiting for the results immediately administered massive doses of antibiotics.

The lab surprisingly found no presence of harmful bacteria. This was extremely puzzling. Baker again inspected the incision, initially a neat six-inch cut, and found more black flesh. Because it is less weakening to the abdominal wall, he had used a Pfannenstiel incision, in which the outer skin and underlying fat are cut horizontally, and spread open, permitting the surgeon to separate to separate the abdominal muscles vertically to reach the uterus.

Not only had the infection spread, but Mrs. Kreuter's fever was worse, spiking to 103 degrees. Baker desperately needed to know what kind of bug was causing the trouble, so he could get the specific antibiotic that would cure the infection. He sent more smears to the laboratory. Still no bugs cultured out, other than some minor yeast organism that does no more than produce an itch.

"She was getting worse by the hour," Baker recalls. "It was really weird. We couldn't understand it. She was getting sick out of proportion to whatever was causing the toxin."

Baker administered a big assortment of antibiotics in hopes of lucking onto the correct one-tetracycline, penicillin, ampicillin, Keflin, and reluctantly one he believes is "very dangerous to use," gentamicin sulfate. The obstetrician was blindly fighting an infection whose identity and full characteristics he didn't know.

Mrs. Kreuter's husband, a young General Electric Company engineer, was frightened, and Baker could offer him no satisfactory explanation, not much reassurance. The doctor didn't know himself precisely what was wrong.

The hospital laboratory made a frantic new effort to identify the bug. Cultures were run on every person who had been present when the twins were delivered, as well as on every piece of equipment in the operating room. All came out negative, while the new mother went steadily downhill. The black area grew in size, and her rotting incision finally burst open! Baker felt even more frustrated and frantic. He kept thinking of another woman who had undergone a Caesarean at Good Samaritan only a few weeks before and who had later developed abscesses and died of the infection.

"I didn't want to lose a mamma," Baker recalls. "I never have. I called in a surgeon and an internal medical specialist for consultation. Mrs. Kreuter's infection was spreading like a forest fire. She was out of her head from the high fever."

In the operating room, the three doctors examined the infected area. It looked terrible. The black flesh now formed a two-inch wide band stretching ten inches across her lower abdomen. They decided to perform standard surgical debridement which means cutting away all the dead and dying flesh, in which bacteria multiply and manufacture toxins that poison the entire body.

Baker was fearful that in the operating room, they would find the infection had invaded her abdominal muscle structure, and possibly the uterus. Fortunately, it had not. Only the skin and its underlying fat layer were diseased.

But this surgery helped little. Two days later the area of infection had widened to six by twelve inches, driving her fever spikes to 105 degrees. It was now clearly a losing battle. Baker knew such infections had a mortality rate of about 60 per cent. The germs had to be stopped, or the new mother might not live another week.

The doctor lay awake at night, racking his brain. What could he do to save Mrs. Kreuter's life? Something vague began ticking in the back of his mind. But it didn't come to him right away.

"We were all desperately trying to come up with something. We were flat stumped. We couldn't culture the bug, but we all had come to the conclusion it had to be some anaerobe, a bug that survives only in the absence of oxygen. Then suddenly it hit me—something Randy Cochran had told me two or three months before."

Randy Cochran had been a friend of Baker's since before the doctor finished Indiana University Medical School in 1964 and is photo director of The Kentucky Post and Times-Star, of which I am editor. This is a Scripps-Howard newspaper in Covington, Kentucky, just across the Ohio River from Cincinnati.

During the months spent researching this book, I had frequently discussed with Randy Cochran the utterly amazing things I was finding about hyperbaric medicine. I also introduced him to Dr. Cornelia Dettmer, head of the Oncology Department at Cincinnati's Christ Hospital. In November 1971, she installed in her department a one-patient Vickers chamber, the only available clinical hyperbaric facility in southwestern Ohio. I had interviewed her for material for the book. Randy Cochran met her in midsummer when he escorted the doctor and her three children on a fossil hunt at Kentucky's famous Big Bone Lick.

"I remembered," Baker says, "that Randy Cochran told me he had met a hyperbaric doctor, a woman. I remembered that because she was a fossil buff, as I am. But I didn't know her name or where her tank was located.

At that moment, Baker had no clear knowledge of hyperbaric therapy. Further, the other doctors trying to save Mrs. Kreuter knew only vaguely about tank treatments. But all agreed it might be good in theory.

A phone call to Randy Cochran put Baker quickly in touch with Dettmer. She was just leaving on vacation. "I'll cancel that," she told Baker. "Bring your patient right over."

Within an hour, Mrs. Kreuter was wheeled into Christ's Hospital's oncology section. Dettmer had her Vickers chamber, a sturdy plastic capsule thirty inches in diameter and seven feet long, ready. Mrs. Kreuter, barely rational, had given up; she thought she would surely die, or if not, the rotting wound would leave her a cripple for life.

Nurses slipped a non-static surgical gown over her, put her on a small stretcher, and pushed it inside, closed and bolted the tank's end cover. Pure oxygen was pumped in and brought to a pressure of two atmospheres, or 29.4 pounds per square inch. In large walk-in chambers, the pressure is obtained by compressing room air, and the patient breathes oxygen by mask. In the small tanks, no mask is necessary, for the whole interior is pressurized with pure oxygen.

Within minutes, the oxygen she was breathing tremendously enriched her blood and began literally "drenching" her whole body. Watching through the transparent canopy of the tank, Dettmer and Baker were elated to see the edges of the gaping wound turned pink and healthy.

Mrs. Kreuter took a two-hour dive, and the treatment was repeated twice daily. On the third day her fever broke!

"From there on out, "Baker recalls, "it was uphill all the way. It was one of the most dramatic turn-arounds in a patient's course I have ever seen. "

Exactly which microbe had invaded her incision was never precisely determined. But it no longer mattered.

A skillful surgeon was able to neatly close the skin over her abdominal defect and Mrs. Kreuter was well enough two weeks later to pose for newspaper photographers at home with her daughters, Kelly and Krista, and her husband.

The thankful patient and her grateful obstetrician were telling their dramatic story to try to help spread the word.

2

MAGIC IN YOUR BLOOD

Anyone who happens to discover the amazing hyperbaric chamber usually asks a couple of quick questions:

Precisely how does the tank work its magic?

If it's all that wonderful, why don't more doctors use it?

There's a straightforward answer for the first question, based on a trio of long-known scientific laws. The second requires a good bit of thoughtful consideration.

Hyperbaric medicine has a surprisingly long history. European Physicians first attempted three hundred years ago to improve human respiration under compressed air. They achieved little, if any, success. Their equipment and understanding then were both inadequate.

In the early 1800s, the therapy was put to rather wide clinical use on a sort of health-spa basis, principally in England and France. This vogue bumbled along, spread across the continent, but finally died out at the end of the 19th century.

Compressed-air tank treatments were again tried in America at the end of World War I but encountered an aggressive challenge from organized medicine. The American Medical Association's mini war on this unconventional treatment clouded the claims made for its effectiveness. Even so, for more than a decade, thousands of sick Americans submitted themselves to hyperbaric oxygenation for a wide variety of disabilities—ranging from diabetes and syphilis to pneumonia and hypertension. The roster of patients included some of the nation's wealthy and famous.

Memories of this bitter and distorted controversy still haunt the world of medicine and seem indirectly responsible for much of the undercurrent of doubt that causes many in the profession to stubbornly cling to the notion that the hyperbaric chamber is an untamed Maverick somehow not to be trusted.

Evidence to the contrary is clear and abundant. The truth is that current treatments are very effective. Yet, it is painfully obvious that even greater proof is needed to restore or establish faith. There is a vast army of unbelievers.

During the last decade, medical journals steadily have reported favorable clinical results from hyperbaric treatment applied to no less than twenty diseases or injury conditions. Thousands of lives have been saved. And in almost every case, death was cheated at the 11th hour after some frustrated doctor already had vainly tried every other trick in his medical bag. The salvaging of Corporal Helfer and Mrs. Kreuter are dramatic typical examples.

Numerous similar cases have been published. Why didn't the doctors who read these accounts become influenced toward a broad acceptance of HBO? The answer is murky. For one thing, many physicians seem to feel built-in negativism toward new wrinkles in medicine they can't grasp quickly. Not warming up to hyperoxygenation, they probably don't discuss it with their patients. This, in turn, tends to keep the layman relatively ignorant, and thus depresses any curiosity he might express about tank treatments.

There's a more practical drawback. Big hyperbaric chambers are cumbersome and expensive; not readily available to the average doctor. Likewise, they require a trained operator, someone with the skills of a Navy Master diver. Even the simpler-to-use one-patient chambers are not accessible in most cities.

By contrast, nowadays even a small-town surgeon could assemble all the operating room devices he would need for a procedure as exotic as a heart transplant more quickly than he can lay hands on a hyperbaric tank.

Many doctors—readily conceding that lives have been saved—consider the overall results of hyperbaric oxygenation erratic, and feel that it is essentially dangerous, too expensive, and not adequately proven. And even today, the idea is tainted and damaged in some circles by the lingering stigma—warranted or not! —that the hyperbaric chamber was commercialized and over-promoted fifty years ago.

For whatever reason it exists, this foot-dragging takes a tragic toll in the nation's health. Sick people are paying the cost in untimely death. Not a day passes on which a patient could not be saved if some doctor had the alertness, the knowledge, or the confidence to put him in a hyperbaric chamber.

A reasonable guesstimate on needless deaths can be postulated from government statistics on merely one of the illnesses known to respond to HBO—carbon monoxide poisoning. This is known as America's most senseless accidental killer. Householders are caught unaware to fumes from faulty heaters and flues or by automobile exhaust in enclosed garages, often while asleep. Workers are also overcome in mines and factories.

One thousand five hundred people die of carbon-monoxide poisoning annually in the United States, and 10,000 suffer chronic ill effects from exposure to the poison.

One expert hazards a guess that 800 to 900 fatalities could be prevented by prompt hyperbaric oxygenation.

If more firemen, ambulance drivers, rescue squadsmen, policemen, and doctors in emergency rooms knew the location of the nearest hyperbaric chamber, many carbon-monoxide victims would have a better chance. Such a system already has been proved out in Milwaukee. And that example could benefit other cities which have magnificent hyperbaric chambers that, ironically, are standing virtually idle, and totally unknown to fire and police squads. Every major city should have at least one tank for this emergency alone.

When many questions about everyday problems of health—such as how to cure the simple cold—still baffle the best medical minds, is it really so unusual that certain mysteries of basic human physiology should create deep conflict in our laboratories and clinics? Certainly not.

Uncertainty about hyperbaric medicine persists in and out of the profession. That is a prime reason for this book. For the first time, in these pages is drawn together the complete account of how this unorthodox and fascinating method of healing originated, how it flourished and faded—

Page not merely once before, but twice; a record that straightens out shameful misconceptions from the past and attempts to fairly and accurately detail both of its golden moments of heroic triumph as well as the full dossier of unvarnished fact on its dismal failures.

The subject is especially timely. The future of hyperbaric medicine in America appears to hang in the balance. Unless greater effort is made to try to capitalize HBO's obvious potential, present apathy presages another gradual descent back into the obscurity of the past.

Future direction largely hinges on whether fresh leadership and financing can be generated to assess the nagging doubts that still cloud the maverick "miracle" tank. Such needed wide-scale testing would be costly, probably so expensive it would be feasible only under direct government sponsorship, in the same manner that virtually all health research for the public's common good is financed.

Even among hyperbarists themselves, controversy flares. Renowned physicians, with equal training and skill, take opposite sides. Some researchers who began eager and bright-eyed ten years ago now are disillusioned, and have shut down their half-million dollar tanks, or rarely use them. Yet at the same time, other still-confident experimenters with meager 27,000-dollar one-patient chambers busily and doggedly persist—and report stunning results.

Medicine seems to be like that. The average layman, who generally stands in awe of the intricacies of this science of healing, must be greatly puzzled by the mechanics of hyperbaric oxygenation, if he knows about it at all. The aim of this book is to enlighten him, to make the whole picture, mechanics and result, clear and understandable.

A good beginning is to answer the primary technical question, hopefully in everyday language. How exactly does hyperbaric oxygenation work its magic? What actually happened to Corporal Helfer and Mrs. Kreuter inside the tanks? Couldn't they have received the same benefit by breathing pure oxygen through a regular face mask or under the usual hospital tent?

First, we should briefly consider the function of our marvelous respiratory system. Normal breathing is so effortless and automatic that we seldom are conscious of it; and a healthy person breathes about 16 times a minute.

Air is composed of about 21% oxygen and about 79% nitrogen (plus traces of such exotic gases as argon, neon, helium, krypton and xenon). Forget about everything except the 21 percent oxygen, which is almost precisely the amount the body normally requires to maintain life.

As we inhale each breath, the air enters the lungs where it is immediately drawn into minute pouches known as the alveoli. There are an incredible number of these microscopic air sacs—400 million. The alveoli walls are lined with a moist, ultrathin membrane that is such a vast surface it could be spread out to cover a tennis court, but instead is amazingly folded and crinkled so that it fits inside the five lobes of the lungs.

Beyond the thin walls of the alveoli are the equally thin-walled capillaries, in which blood is flowing. Both these walls are semi-permeable, and the oxygen-gas molecules pass through them and combine with the gas molecules in the bloodstream. To understand the enormous and delicate complexity of this mechanism, it is worth knowing that the total length of the capillaries in the lungs has been calculated at 1,000 miles.

So the oxygen breathed in readily diffuses into the blood which transports it systematically to individual cells in all parts of the body. These cells, of course, require this oxygen to create energy, and in exchange, release resulting wastewater, heat, and carbon dioxide into the veins to be carried back to the lungs and exhaled.

Your outgoing breath is made up of just about as much nitrogen as you inhaled (nitrogen is actually not required by the body but seems to serve a useful purpose in providing the bulk that keeps the lungs inflated) and about 150 times more carbon dioxide, most of it "exhaust" from the cells' energy-making "workshops." Then your next breath starts the cycle all over again.

In normal circumstances, oxygen is transported in the blood only by the hemoglobin in the red blood cells. Oxygen molecules have such an affinity for the red cells that the hemoglobin is always about 97 or 98 percent saturated with oxygen. A fact of great importance in hyperbaric medicine is that the red cells constitute only 45% of our blood volume; and that the other 55%, the colorless plasma, transports hardly any oxygen at all.

This imbalance between the workload of the red cells and the plasma is precisely what makes possible the magic of HBO. But to understand how it comes about, you must consider the weight and degree of atmospheric pressure in which we live. Hyperbaric literally means high pressure. If we are living at sea level, we are under one atmosphere of pressure absolute, which can also be expressed as 760 millimeters of mercury (mm. Hg), 29.9 inches Mercury, or, 14.7 pounds per square inch.

You don't feel or notice this normal pressure because it is all balanced, the same amount of pressure is exerted inside your body, on and in the organs, and on the blood and on the oxygen in the air you breathe.

Long ago, physicians speculated that a person who suffered a hypoxic or ischemic illness in which body tissues literally starve for oxygen ought to be somehow forced to breathe in more oxygen. Why not inhale pure 100% oxygen instead of the regular air containing 21% oxygen? That sounded like a winner, and it was tried. It didn't help much the reason was that the red cells already carrying 97 to 98% of their capacity could only take on two or three percent more oxygen while the plasma continued to run virtually empty.

That was that—until somebody began considering scientific laws governing the behavior of gases. Boyle's law states that the pressure of a given quantity of gas whose temperature remains unchanged varies inversely as its volume. That means that if you desire to double the pressure of a gas within a container, twice the amount of gas must be forced into the chamber. Into a modern large hyperbaric chamber can be forced as much as six times the amount of gas—therefore, resulting in six times the amount of pressure—that it would contain when the chamber interior is at normal atmospheric pressure.

Another law, Dalton's, holds that the total pressure exerted by a mixture of gases is equal to the sum of the partial pressures of the individual gases. Thus, at sea level nitrogen exerts a partial pressure of about 600 (mm. Hg) and oxygen about 760 (mm. Hg). If the total pressure of air is doubled, as it can be in a hyperbaric tank, the percentage of nitrogen and oxygen in the air will remain the same but the partial pressure of each gas will be doubled.

The amount of a slightly soluble gas such as oxygen that can be dissolved in a solution in contact with the gas is directly proportional to the partial pressure of the gas. This is Henry's law.

What the application of these three laws in essence means is that if the partial pressure of oxygen in contact with alveolar capillaries is increased, there will be a corresponding increase in the amount of oxygen that will be forced into solution in the blood. And about the only place this extra oxygen can go is into the previously "empty" plasma.

Thus, when the pressure in a hyperbaric chamber is increased from the normal one atmosphere (sea level) to 3 atmospheres the partial pressure of oxygen will be increased from 160 to 480 mm. Hg (Dalton's law).

Henry's law says the amount of oxygen forced into solution in the blood would go up correspondingly; but just how much?

The increase is phenomenal. If the patient is breathing ordinary air inside the hyperbaric chamber under pressure of 3 atmospheres absolute, the partial pressure of oxygen in the arteries will jump to over 400 mm. Hg, a gain in the blood oxygen content of about 1.7 volumes per cent.

Let the patient instead breathe 100% oxygen at 3 atmospheres absolute and the arterial blood will zoom to 1,720 mm. Hg, an increase in oxygen content of 6.1 volumes per cent!

This is a sensational increase in the oxygen going into the blood. A comparison that dramatically illustrates the point is this: when the body is in resting condition, it normally consumes only about 6 milliliters of oxygen per 100 milliliters of blood. Of this only about 0.3 milliliters of the oxygen is transported by the plasma.

But hyperbaric pressure raised to three times normal increases the plasma's oxygen content to 6.6 milliliters—or more than enough for the body's total needs at rest without counting oxygen normally in the hemoglobin.

Under triple pressure, the amount of oxygen in the hyperbaric patient's blood thus is increased to ten to fifteen times normal!

Thus, the hyperbaric chamber can make the difference between life and death for a desperately ill patient whose diseased or injury-whacked body must have an above normal oxygen supply.

Tanks in use range from single-patient models about seven feet long and about 30 inches in diameter (resembling an iron lung in size) to giants about as big as a railroad tank car, roughly 12 feet in diameter by 50 feet in length, large enough to contain a complete operating room setup. Hyperbaric physicians have acquired most of their terminology from deep-sea divers, who made the first major use of compressed air.

Pressure in the tanks is measured in units of atmospheres absolute, abbreviated as ATA. The reading at sea level, of course, is 1 ATA, which is equivalent to 760 mm. Hg, Or expressed another way 14.7 pounds per square inch. And beyond the 1 ATA which is present at sea level, each atmosphere is equivalent to the pressure exerted by 33 feet of sea water.

This table shows how those measurements compare:

ATA	mm Hg	Psia	Ft.	sea depth
1	760	14.7	0	(sea level)
2	1520	29.4	33	
3	2280	44.1	66	
4	3040	58.8	99	
5	4800	73.5	132	
6	5560	88.2	165	

In most hyperbaric chambers, treatments are given at three ATA, which is equivalent to a pressure of 2,280 millimeters of mercury, or 44.1 pounds per square inch, or what a diver would feel at a depth of 66 feet below the surface of the sea. In most hyperbaric chambers, treatments are given at three ATA, which is equivalent to a pressure of 2,280 millimeters of mercury, or 44.1 pounds per square inch, or what a diver would feel at a depth of 66 feet below the surface of the sea.

3

LE BAIN D'AIR COMPRIME

The first medical use of a hyperbaric chamber was undertaken three centuries ago in England by a Dr Henshaw. That seems incredible. Henshaw couldn't have known much about what he was doing. It was fully one hundred years before oxygen was to be discovered!

Physicians in the 1600s still were really quite ignorant about chemistry, physiology, and even anatomy. They were just beginning to question the prevailing ancient Galen theory of respiration which identified the heart as the body's heat generator. Second-century Greek physician Claudius Galen thought man breathed air only to cool his fiery heart, exhaling its smoky vapors. That was said to explain why animals died in air-tight vessels—they couldn't cool themselves.

In such unenlightened climate, the intrepid Henshaw in 1662 rigged a large pair of organ bellows to pump air into a closed room he called a "domicilium." What triggered his brainstorm is not recorded, but he was way ahead of his time. He arranged his valves to either compress or rarefy the air inside the chamber, a nifty feature of sum of today's tanks. His technical know-how had to be woefully inadequate. How did he seal his room? It couldn't have been airtight enough to hold much above normal sea level pressure; and it is laughable to imagine his bellows creating sufficient partial vacuum to effectively lower pressure.

His rationale for providing a choice of atmospheres was interesting. Elevated pressures, he allowed, should help acute diseases, low pressure the chronic conditions. Somehow his agile mind may have zeroed in on the fact that seashore and mountain climbs offered therapeutic benefits—for precisely opposite reasons.

Henshaw imagined he had discovered a stunning panacea. To quote him, "In time of good health, this domicilium is proposed as a good expedient to help digestion, to promote insensible respiration, to facilitate breathing and expectoration, and consequently, of excellent use for the prevention of most affections of the lungs."

Give the good doctor credit for a pioneering shot in the dark, but Henshaw's contraption must have failed miserably. If the domicilium did achieve sensational clinical results, the records have somehow been misplaced. What must have even been worse for his ego, Henshaw didn't even inspire competition. It was about two hundred years before the next doctor cranked up a hyperbaric chamber.

All the while, of course, man was daring the deep and the exploits of those hesitant early divers were being inextricably woven into the fabric of HBO history because each splash contributed a little to technical advances, as they still do.

For centuries, the breath-holding alone acquired what might be called hyperbaric experience. The pearl and sponge divers in the Mediterranean and Indian and Pacific Oceans relied on fantastic lungs. But finally, some less hearty soul stumbled upon the diving-bell principle. Alexander the Great of Macedonia is said to have descended into the sea for a prolonged period in a barrel made from glass and animal skins. This gave him a secret weapon in his siege of Tyre (332 B.C.).

It required another nineteen hundred years for the state of the diving art to advance to upending a big kettle and suspending it below the surface by ropes. Two Greeks, in the trapped airspace of such a diving bell, descended in 1538 to the bottom of the Tagus. One pop-eyed observer of their safe ascent was Charles V of Spain.

And the physicians, puttering away in their laboratories, had not yet got around to discovering oxygen or carbon dioxide, or learning the why of blood circulation.

But oddly enough, right at the time Henshaw's big bellows were wheezing away, the Dutch tried to invent the submarine. That gave 17th-century skeptics a good laugh—but not hapless the Dutch sailors swallowing sea water.

Nearly a century later, the French too gave it a more successful try, experimenting with their first sub in 1749. And in 1775 (just to show how many years all this took) a Yale graduate, David Bushnell, built for General George Washington an egg-shaped submarine made principally of iron-ringed barrel staves. Its mission was to sneak up under British warships in New York harbor and screw explosives to their bottoms. Called The Turtle, the sub proved seaworthy and was able to move around pretty well with its hand-cranked propeller. But The Turtle encountered all manner of bad luck, barely eluded capture—and never blew up any Man o' war invaders.

Meanwhile, 18th-century researchers got busy and expanded the frontiers in chemistry and physiology. Scottish chemist-anatomist Joseph Black discovered carbon dioxide in 1757, and nine years later, English chemist Henry Cavendish found hydrogen. The really significant breakthrough came in 1771 when a 38 year-old English clergyman-chemist, Joseph Priestley, discovered oxygen.

Everybody was still pretty much hoodwinked at the time by that false fiery heart theory. So even Priestley's ideas about respiration were somewhat confused. Thinking in terms of inflammability, he called oxygen the phlogistication of dephlogisticated air. In truth, phlogisticated air was nitrogen and dephlogisticated air was oxygen.

Yet Priestley's classic description of his scientific Everest showed rare insight into the distant future:

"From the greater strength and vivacity of a candle in this pure air, it may be conjectured that it might be peculiarly salutary to the lungs in certain morbid cases...But, perhaps we may also infer from these experiments, that though pure dephlogisticated air might be very useful as a medicine, it might not be so proper for us in the usual healthy state of the body: for as a candle burns out much faster in dephlogisticated then in common air, so we might, as may be said, live out too fast and the animal powers be too soon exhausted in this pure kind of air. A moralist, at least, may say that the air which nature has provided for us is as good as we deserve...The feeling of it in my lungs is not sensibly different from that of common air; but I fancied that my breast felt peculiarly light and easy for some time afterwards. Who could tell but that, in time, this pure air may become a fashionable article of luxury. Hitherto only two mice and myself have had the privilege of breathing it."

Priestley's achievement fired the imagination, but not the energies, of his medical contemporaries. Most of the old guard seemed content to merely speculate on its importance both as a cause and as a cure for many diseases.

It remained for Thomas Beddoes, an eleven-year-old Shropshire lad at the time oxygen was discovered, to grow up and exploit its use medically. Curious and brilliant, Beddoes studied medicine at Edinburgh, lectured in chemistry for five years at Oxford, went to Paris where he met the great Antoine Laurent Lavoisier and, unfortunately burned his fingers meddling in pre-French Revolution politics.

Returning home in the 1780s, Beddoes established the pneumatic laboratory at Bristol, where he demonstrated that inhalation of air heavily enriched with pure oxygen was helpful in a dozen or so illnesses. These range, he wrote perhaps too optimistically from scrofulous affections and asthma to paralysis and leprosy.

James Watt, engineer and inventor of the steam engine, gave Beddoes a hand designing equipment for his experiments. What a super-hyperbaric chamber these two great minds could have produced; but there is no indication they ever discussed it. What undoubtedly helped devise Beddoes' ingenious breathing bags and face masks which were made of oiled silk and attached to a wooden valve box fitted with inspiratory and expiratory check valves.

All this experimenting with oxygen might have been expected to excite interest in hyperbaric medicine. But it didn't. Trying to motivate inventive minds, the Dutch Academy of Sciences offered a prize from 1782 through 1791 for the design of an apparatus to study the effect of high pressures on biology. Not even one gadget was submitted.

Almost half a century was yet to pass before the first hyperbaric craze burst forth. In the interim, underwater man was advancing his know-how. An improved diving bell was used by the English in 1788 to make repairs on bridge underpinning in the River Tyne at Hexham, Northumberland. What made this model so super was it somebody decided to supply the bell with air through a hose connected to a surface pump! That made the next step pretty obvious, and in England in 1819 August Siebe took it; he invented the suit we associate with deep sea divers—the helmet and hose permitting free and daring movement underwater.

Next came the caisson, which enabled man to excavate in harbors and tunnels, bringing an immediate by-product, the mysterious bends. The caisson was a cofferdam into which workmen descended through airlocks into a compressed air chamber. It was the invention of French engineers and Triger scored a first in 1841 by sinking a caisson sixty-five-feet through quicksand to the bed of the Loire River.

In the early 1830s, France suddenly went wild about hyperbaric therapy. Chambers sprang up in half a dozen cities. Physicians dubbed this therapeutic regimen, compressed air baths—*le bain d'air comprime*. Health-seekers flock to the pressurized tanks expecting benefits akin to those derived from mineral water spas.

The first to go into business was a Dr. Junod. One bright morning in 1834, with a roll of drawings under his arm, he strolled into a Paris ironmongers' shop and asked if they could rivet together a copper sphere precisely five feet in diameter fitted with appropriate glass portals, a door that would seal tight, and provide air supply and exhaust connections. The odd metalsmith calculated that he could, struck a price, and started hammering copper sheets.

For those times, Junod was quite sophisticated in his concept of machinery, methods, and aims. He pumped into this copper ball enough air to reach levels similar to those in wide use today—pressures of 2, 2.5, and 4 atmospheres absolute.

Inside the chamber, his grateful patients invariably experienced a sense of well- being. Junod postulated this resulted from improved cerebral blood flow, and he guessed that all internal organs were somehow getting a richer blood supply. He was entirely correct.

The craze spread in 1837 to Lyon where a Dr. Pravaz promptly demonstrated imagination and great faith. He built a big chamber, one that accommodated a dozen patients at a time. It was the largest chamber of that decade.

Pravaz attempted cures on an astonishing assortment of ailments. Into his chamber trooped patients with whooping cough, deafness, uterine bleeding, cholera, rickets, and tracheitis, or worse. He reported a number of successful treatments in the Bulletin of the Académie of Medicine (Paris).

During the next 40 years, the fame of hyperbaric therapy spread rapidly over Western Europe, resulting in construction of scores of pneumatic centers—in Berlin, Stockholm, Amsterdam, Brussels, London, Vienna, and Milan, and elsewhere. Patients were attracted from even America, and someone in Oshawa, Canada took the hint and built there in 1860 the first North American chamber.

In this period, the Civil War broke out in America. Militarists of the South poured over Europe's most recent pressure chamber and diving technology for helpful hints on designing an attack submarine.

The Confederates removed the boiler from a Mississippi stern wheeler and hammered it into a 30-foot long cigar-shaped sub, hand-propelled by a crew of nine. Christened the C.S.S. Hunley, it promptly sank on the trial run, drowning all hands. Salvaged and revamped, it sank again with a crew of nine. It was raised once more, tinkered with, and finally sent into battle.

Carrying a ninety-pound charge of gunpowder lashed to its bow, with a delayed-action fuse, the Hunley sneaked out of Charleston, South Carolina at dusk February 17th, 1864, to attack the Yankee Ironclad Housatonic, which had the city blockaded. Just outside the harbor entrance, the Hunley blew up, killing the crew. The Housatonic also took a mortal wound, listed and slowly sank, with a loss of five federal seamen. Somehow the unleashed charge meant to be left stuck near the enemy's warship keel while the sub beat a safe retreat—had gone off prematurely.

At about the same time, the French built the first power-driven submarine, the 140-foot Plongeur. Her hull was of iron and curiously enough, the propellers were driven by a compressed air motor.

In Europe, research and clinical interests remain high in HBO. Physicians were destined to get an interest-dampening scare further down the road, but first the hyperbaric chamber achieved a new and greater status; it was converted into an operating room. This was done in France in the late 1870s by Dr J. A. Fontaine. He had the foresight to put the whole contraption on wheels, with a manually operated compressor, to make it mobile, pointing out that "with this chamber, one can do surgery in hospitals, sanitaria, and private homes."

In a three-month period, twenty-seven operations were done in the portable tank. A noted Paris surgeon, Jules Emile Péan, did the surgery with five or six assistants. They couldn't have felt cramped; the chamber would accommodate ten to twelve people. These patients were said to have experienced quicker recovery from anesthetics, with no cyanosis or asphyxia, less vomiting, etc.

This success was so impressive, Fontaine wrote two books about this new therapy and drew plans for a pressurized operating theater that would hold three hundred. It was never built, perhaps because Fontaine was HBO's first physician-martyr. An American medical historian attributes Fontaine's death to an accident at his pneumatic center but cites no date. I found no Paris medical historian who could verify the story.

The European hyperbaric surge was reaching a crest. All manner of diseases had been treated; and even singers tried intermittent dives to strengthen their voices. But the noted French physiologist Paul Bert in his busy laboratory unmasked dark side effects of oxygen and became quite perturbed.

Bert was experimenting with oxygen on plants as well as larks and dogs. His tests involved varying combinations of oxygen enrichment. He applied and lifted pressure both slowly and rapidly, and often held animals in its squeeze for long hours.

Bert saw rapid decompression release nitrogen bubbles into the blood where they could block circulation. His larks could not live more than a few minutes in pure oxygen. His thin small dog survived the usually fatal decompressions after experimental dives to 7 and 8 ATA. But when fattened and subjected to a rerun of this test, the dog died, indicating solubility values of nitrogen in fat had to be reckoned with carefully. Oxygen...very toxic! Bert's discoveries ran up the first caution flag, warning that oxygen toxicity hazards should be guarded against and further explored.

This alert was especially disconcerting to the new fraternity of caisson engineers because in the very year of Bert's warning—1879—underwater pier excavations were begun in Antwerp as well as in New York City for the Brooklyn Bridge.

The mysterious bends already was a menace to sandhogs. Some of these laborers, after working six or seven hours down inside the compressed air chamber, felt severe pain in arms and knees shortly after climbing the ladder to the open air. They did not yet know that this was caused by the nitrogen bubbles Bert observed, and that precise tables for slow decompression had to be formulated, and that the bends could prove fatal. (It was not even dreamed, of course, that in this modern era scuba and professional divers would be frequently treated for accidental bends in gleaming 300,000-dollar hyperbaric chambers.)

By 1885, most of the zest had vanished from hyperbaric work in Europe; and far across the ocean in Odell, Nebraska, lived five-year-old Orval J. Cunningham, who was early in the 20th century to put his heavy and indelible imprint on an American revival of *le bain d'air comprime*.

It is not at all difficult to ascertain the reason for the demise of the pneumatic centers in Europe. They were simply oversold. A conservative clinician of the time had warned: "the confidence this treatment deserves might be lost by overemphasizing its value."

Yet the optimistic and ambitious physicians kept reaching for the miracle therapy they were never able to deliver.

A present-day authority of hyperbaric history, Dr. Nicholas G. Meijne, the Amsterdam surgeon who helped pioneer the notable Dutch upsurge at HBO, sums up the era of the European pneumatic chambers this way:

It seems very likely that there was a definite value in the treatment in the pneumatic centers. Notwithstanding that the extra amount of oxygen given by air under pressure, usually 2 to 3 ATA, was very small and even less than when oxygen at 1 ATA would have been given, the physiological effects have certainly been great.

Some authorities of that period lamented the failure of their medical profession to continue experiments in hope of extracting more rewarding benefits from pressurization. Next slide writing in the British medical journal of 1885, Dr C. Theodore Williams of the Brompton Hospital observed:

"The use of atmospheric air under different degrees of atmospheric pressure in the treatment of disease is one of the most important advances in modern medicine, when we considered the simplicity of the agent, the exact methods by which it may be applied, and the precision by which it can be regulated to the requirements of each individual, we are astonished that in England this method of treatment has been so little used."

The HBO bubble had, nonetheless, burst on that side of the Atlantic.

In 1889, Sir Ernest Moir came to New York City to design and build the first medical airlock to decompress Hudson River tunnel workers who were being stricken by the bends.

Sandhogs were required by the contractors to follow a routine decompression schedule; but no one yet had clear understanding of the dangerous and uncertain physiological impact of prolonged pressurization. Reactions differed greatly among individual workers, typical of erratic responses which even today complicate hyperbaric treatments. A further problem was that many early sandhogs, generally a hearty daredevil breed, often were too impatient to tediously sit out full decompression time. So, caisson disease persisted.

Digging the East River tunnels for the Pennsylvania Railroad, according to the medical directors' report in 1909, produced 3,692 cases of decompression sickness—of which 20 were fatal.

At the time of that report, Dr Orval J. Cunningham was five years beyond graduation from Chicago's noted Rush Medical College and destiny was fitting to him a long and controversial shadow that still actively spans five decades to significantly touch present-day developments in hyperbaric medicine.

4

DAUNTLESS DR. CUNNINGHAM

In 1918, an influenza epidemic swept across the United States. Doctors found themselves almost helpless, with no effective medicine (this was long before discovery of antibiotic drugs) or treatment to conquer the disease. A shuddering toll was predicted, half a million lives lost, counting the Americans in khaki in waning World War 1.

The dilemma challenged the imagination of a doctor in Kansas City, Missouri–Dr Orval J. Cunningham, an internist and anesthesiologist aged 38. After mulling it over, he was struck that September by brilliant inspiration.

The germ of his idea had come to him four months previously during a vacation trip to Colorado. Looking down 1,053 feet into the Royal Gorge, Cunningham reflected on the fact that mortality and pneumonia is greater at high altitudes, where the air pressure is lower. Also, in the mountains there was a greater prevalence of rheumatism, neuritis, heart disease, and high blood pressure. Doctors found patients with these ills usually improved when sent to lower altitudes; they got more oxygen out of the air they breathe because of the higher pressure of the atmosphere at sea level.

Cunningham had observed that flu victims in Kansas City died cyanotic—blue and starved for oxygen. It struck him that he could create a controlled environment of artificial high pressure for them. He reviewed the writing of famed French physiologist Paul Bert, and decided to employ a large, compressed air tank.

He patterned his sketch along the lines of a caisson workers' decompression chamber, 10 by 30 feet, entered through hatches and an airlock. It could accommodate a doctor and three or four patients and was no amateur design. Cunningham had a keen engineering mind. He had built gas mixing machines to give more effective anesthesia and was admired by the surgeons in Kansas City hospitals for his technical skill and diagnostic brilliance.

In spare moments, he tinkered with a design for a new-type internal combustion motor; he was trying to marry the two-cycle and four-cycle principles. He also was attempting to slow down sound so a stethoscope could detect the precise click of valves opening and closing in the heart.

In mid-October, he presented his tank design to Dr. M. F. Sudler, dean of the fledgling Kansas University Medical School just across the Missouri River on "Goat Hill" in suburban Rosedale, Kansas. In addition to his private practice, Cunningham was K.U.'s professor of anesthesiology.

The dean and Dr. C. F. Nelson, professor of chemistry, were quite impressed. Cunningham postulated that the compressed air tanks increased oxygenation might be also effective against anaerobic infections. Sudler and Nelson saw some merit in that speculation.

Cunningham proposed building the tank near one of the Goat Hill buildings to be used as a research tool, and Sudler went along with that idea. On October 24, 1918, the dean dispatched a letter to Chancellor Strong on the main campus at Lawrence, Kansas, stating that Cunningham wished to try compressed air on flu patients, and that the medical faculty was in accord, provided he first did experimental work in the device with rabbits.

Cunningham knew precisely what he needed. For days, he prowled the "bottoms" at Kansas City where were clustered grimy machine shops, pipe and junk yards, boilermakers. He spent endless hours on the phone, too. Footing the expense himself, Cunningham cajoled bargain prices, and some credit. Trucks began delivering a myriad collection of metal junk to Goat Hill.

Finally on a sunny afternoon not long after the armistice, the last joint of pipe was coupled and a secondhand boiler from the stockyards had been converted into a compressed-air tank eight feet in diameter and twenty-four feet long. The used compressor thumped and hissed. There were two sections, an entry airlock, and the main chamber, with glass portals welded into the side of the tank. Cunningham and Professor Nelson, a close friend, started up the compressor. The gauge was set for twenty pounds of extra pressure, or about 2.5 ATA. The needle hung right on twenty—no leaks!

But the elated smile froze on Cunningham's face; through the porthole, he saw smoky mist forming thin clouds inside the chamber. The compressor was leaking oil into the air intake. Cunningham spent four or five days dismantling the compressor, polishing the cylinder walls and installing new rings. That fixed the trouble.

Laboratory animals—monkeys, guinea pigs, rabbits—were to be the first "patients." But it didn't work out that way. A doctor stopped Cunningham as he walked out of Bell Memorial Hospital and requested use of the tank. Many Kansas City physicians knew about the contraption, but seemed only mildly interested, if at all. However, this doctor was frustrated because a young friend was dying of pneumonia, and no medicine had helped.

Cunningham was hesitant; he hadn't yet run his animal studies. He examined the patient and saw he might not live four hours. There was no time to debate the matter; so, the young man was rushed to Goat Hill and put into the tank on a makeshift wooden bunk covered with an Army blanket.

The youth's lips already were blue-black and he was deeply unconscious. Cunningham heard air start hissing into the chamber, felt the rise and temperature and humidity, swallowed to make his ears pop and put his stethoscope on the patient's chest. The heart was galloping; his respiration was ragged and brutal; the death rattle could sound at any moment.

Cunningham let the pressure build up by about 10 pounds, not quite 2 ATA, and held it there. He had to feel his way; he dredged his memory for Paul Bert's decompression calculations—coming out of the dive by stages so as not to cause the bends would be the chief danger. He began calculating how long to keep the man in the tank.

Of a sudden, the patient stirred. Cunningham looked and was amazed. The lad's eyes were open, he was turning pink; he was out of his coma. In a few minutes, his heart rate fell ten beats... then fifteen. His fight to suck in each desperate breath got easier. The tank was definitely helping him. Cunningham continued that treatment for a little over an hour. Then, intermittently during the next three days, he gave the patient additional dives. Other doctors could see the pneumonia victim was starting to recover. Obviously, the extra oxygen going into his blood was making the difference. Cunningham was elated. But this hurried action had bypassed the requirement for animal tests before any experiment with humans, and some faculty noses were out of joint.

Yet a few days later, another more abundant pneumonia patient was rushed to Goat Hill. Again the tank and Cunningham saved a life. This successful repeat stirred a vision and Cunningham's mind–this mighty new instrument could bring thousands back to health, and he must do something about it.

One evening, he told his wife Grace he had arranged to buy a big house at 3310 Harrison Avenue and planned to build there a much larger tank, outfitted for his patient's comfort like a Pullman car. A lawyer-friend, B. P. Bagby, was lending him $70,000, secured by a mortgage on the property.

The new tank was an incongruity in the side yard on Harrison Avenue, nestling close to the three-story brick frame house that had a steep gabled roof and many windows overlooking the tree lined street. The heavy steel tank was ten feet in diameter and eighty-eight feet long. There were twenty-four portholes equally spaced along each side, giving it some resemblance to a modern jetliner's exterior. The tank was set about three feet above ground on brick piers and was entered via a wooden ramp through a central airlock that gave onto large chambers in both ends.

These twin compartments were identical, outfitted with seats along the wall that let down like Pullman beds. In each chamber, thirty-six patients could move about freely, and use the showers and toilets. A new building in the rear yard housed electric motors with 160 horsepower to compress 2,000 cubic feet of air per minute and provide 72-degree air conditioning and 65% humidity. This was an enormous improvement over the Goat Hill tank in which summer temperatures were over 100 degrees. Inside the Harrison Avenue house, Cunningham converted rooms into an office and laboratories. He employed a dietitian and cooks and sent meals via heated cart to patients in the tank.

After his success in treating flu and pneumonia, Cunningham had pitted the Goat Hill tank against a variety of chronic illnesses, many of them lung diseases, emphysema, bronchial asthma and other conditions that restrict the body's intake and absorption of oxygen. He also found the dives effective in heart disease, hypertension, acute rheumatic fever, arthritis, and diabetes mellitus, as well as syphilis. (This was prior to the discovery of penicillin.)

Dr. C. C. Dennie, an admirer and a leading Kansas City physician, said in his memoirs, years later:

"Obviously compression of the air increase the oxygen content of the blood. So, it would be natural that his hypertension patients would improve because the tank really takes a load off the heart. I saw patients with hypertension and arthritis improve rapidly."

Word of the Goat Hill tank had spread far beyond Kansas City, so when the Cunningham Sanitarium on Harrison Avenue opened in April 1920, a growing stream of sick people came from many states, some from California,

One of his most talked-about treatments was for diabetes mellitus. Cunningham believed that nearly all diabetes was caused by changes in the pancreas due to toxins of infective origin. His microscope would not single out any one guilty germ, but he was certain it wasn't anaerobe. His treatment may not have been scientifically sound in the light of today's knowledge; but many of his patients who had advanced cases of diabetes returned to their normal weight, were on a full diet, no sugar in the blood, normal blood sugar levels, and all symptoms of the disease gone.

There was no doubt in his mind that the tank was devastating against syphilis. Records of patients with venereal disease were stringently coded, but any medically trained eye could interpret the reference to lues, locomotor, ataxia, tabes dorsalis on blood tests. In a medical journal article on his work, he reported:

"The spirochete (germ) of syphilis is highly anaerobic and can survive (except for short periods) only under anaerobic conditions. Hereditary syphilis seems to respond to the treatment as well as the acquired...the pains of neural-syphilis promptly cease under the treatment with the exception of an occasional case in which some pain is due to the actual enmeshing of nerve fibers in scar tissue."

A peculiar action of this treatment is a marked effect in the regeneration of nerve fibers. After the cell bodies of the nerves are dead, there can be no regeneration, but it seems that there is a degeneration of the nerve fibers long before the death of the cell bodies, and it is the nerves in this condition that return to normal.

Of the first 175 syphilis patients who completed five months of treatment, Cunningham found only two who did not maintain a negative Wasserman test, and one he termed a re-infection and the other probably a laboratory error. His professional colleagues in Kansas City had to be impressed by the caliber of his results, but they did not embrace his compressed-air therapy, and this stung Cunningham.

His attitude about the sanitarium became very guarded. Denny, a sincere friend, later wrote that Cunningham was "very suspicious of anyone who visited the tank other than the patients because he was afraid his secret would be stolen from him."

Merre Shane of Kansas City, a young nurse who worked in the tank, recalled in a 1972 interview that Cunningham "had the busiest brain" of anyone she worked with. "He was much too evasive about what his theory really was, and he was afraid that someone would take advantage of him. But this is true in the history of all wizards and mental giants."

For all its newness, the tank was a calm fixture. Surprisingly, the engine room did not disturb the neighborhood tranquility, though it occasionally ran non-stop for days. In another of his rare medical journal articles, Cunningham gave this description of the tank's operation:

"The time of the treatments varies from two to ten hours of each 24 or 48 hours. In the greater number of cases, it is two or three hours, with air pressure up from five to twenty pounds per square inch above atmospheric pressure depending upon the disease treated and the condition of the patient."

During day treatments, patients wear their street clothes and spend the time visiting, reading, games, or sleeping as they choose. Twenty pounds of pressure a square inch above the surrounding atmospheric pressure, which is the pressure usually employed, would be equivalent to placing the patient in a valley about 26,000 feet, or nearly five miles, below sea level, if that were possible.

Treatments begin at regularly appointed hours. As the pressure is increased during the next few minutes, the patients yawn occasionally, in order to equalize the pressure on both sides of the eardrums. There is nothing disagreeable about the treatment, and under proper methods, no harm can come from it.

Extensive reading had made Cunningham aware of what he termed the "meager experimentation" in the physiological effects of compressed-air treatment, and in deep-sea diving, and especially in prevention of caisson disease, the bends. He told Grace his work in the sanitarium was opening new doors in medicine. The cost in those years of manufacturing oxygen made it too expensive except for limited hospital use. Yet, at nominal cost, his patients were inhaling compressed air that was 60% richer in oxygen than the normal atmosphere of the tank. Further, he told his wife, using compressed air to kill certain bacteria was totally new.

Cunningham considered himself highly ethical and did not advertise. Reporters from the Kansas City Star and the Times pretty much ignored the tank; for some reason, it just wasn't news. But the word spread anyhow, primarily from pleased patients, and business boomed.

The Saturday Evening Post published a half-page photograph of Cunningham's new tank in the issue of March 5th, 1921, to illustrate a long article called "Everybody's Business—What's Next in Science?" Floyd W. Parsons wrote:

"In view of the amazing achievements of man during the past decade, it is no wonder that scientists today are showing a boldness of imagination that must doubtless startle many of the older and more conservative chemical and physical investigators."

One reason why the future is bright lies in the fact that time slowly, but surely removes the reactionaries who block the progress of civilization by belittling invention and by refusing to substitute new ways for old.

Most great discoveries were accidental, and the majority of them were delayed being put into practical use by the skepticism, not of the ignorant, but of famous leaders of contemporary thought. The development of the airplane was retarded by the widely circulated opinion of a noted geologist, who pointed out that man never need expect to fly in a comparatively heavy, power-propelled machine, because of certain definite facts he had discovered relating to the maximum sizes of fossil birds...

Dozens of other epical discoveries might be traced back through the centuries to the patient research work of early experimenters, and yet the adaptation of many of these important inventions to useful service did not occur hundreds of years later...One of the most remarkable developments of recent times is the thought of using compressed air in the treatment of diseases that respond to increased oxidation. In Kansas, (Author's Note: actually, in Kansas City, Missouri), here is an installation of this kind that costs more than one hundred thousand dollars. The apparatus is called The Tank, and consists of a steel cylinder enclosure, eighty-eight feet long and ten feet in diameter. It is equipped with airlocks, toilets, common shower baths, compartments and Pullman-Car equipment...

In the past, people whose health demanded more oxygen have been directed to go to the seashore or to low altitudes, where the barometric pressure is greater. Now, with a development of this new use of compressed air, it appears that we may enjoy all the benefits of a change in altitude without leaving the boundaries of our hometowns...

Nowhere did The Saturday Evening Post write-up mention Dr. Cunningham by name, possibly because he asked that his identity be omitted.

Lawyer Bagby, not only believed in Cunningham's genius enough to back him with $70,000 but tried to persuade a number of national personalities to take advantage of the tank. One such was Franklin D, Roosevelt, just after he had been stricken by crippling infantile paralysis, and a decade before he was elected President.

On the letterhead of Emmett, Marvin & Roosevelt, Counselors at Law, 52 Wall Street, New York City, but sent from Hyde Park, N.Y., on November 17th, 1922, Roosevelt wrote:

"My dear Mr. Bagby:

Many thanks for your very clear letter in regard to Dr Cunningham's aero-therapeutic treatments. I am very much interested in what you write, and it certainly sounds as if Dr. Cunningham has worked out something which is practical and full of common sense in relation to the treatment of many troubles.

Frankly, I have no idea of whether it would or would not be of real benefit in my case. I am suffering from a perfectly normal, but well-defined case of infantile paralysis contracted in August 1921. The symptoms were the usual ones, and though I was not affected above the waist in any way, both legs were put out of commission.

I have been under the care of Dr. Lovett of Boston, who, in the East, is recognized as the greatest authority on infantile paralysis. Under his treatment, I did nothing for the first five or six months—or until the soreness had disappeared from the muscles. Since that time, I've been taking leg and foot muscle exercises prescribed by him. Gradually, but surely the muscles have been coming back, and practically all of them are working to a greater or less extent. This summer, I have been swimming and find that in the water, with the weight taken off, my legs function extremely well. The knees are still too weak to bear my weight, and I am therefore compelled to use leg braces and crutches in order to get about.

Of course, I have no idea of the exact condition of the nerve tissues in the spine at the present time. My general health is extremely good—never better, in fact—and I have no idea what effect an additional portion of oxygen would have..."

Roosevelt never was a patient in the tank. At her California home in the spring of 1972, Mrs. Cunningham, a cultured and spry octogenarian, told me that her husband responded to the letter, advising Roosevelt that the compressed-air therapy would be unlikely to improve his paralytic condition.

In the 20s, the "beautiful people" had no jet planes, but they favored the luxury and speed of the Twentieth Century Limited.

One evening as the sleek train thundered at seventy-five miles an hour across northern Ohio towards Chicago, the two-fisted president of the mighty Remington Rand Corporation entered the club car and joined three other wealthy men at bridge. During the conversation, one mentioned The Tank. A Mrs. Reynolds of St. Louis had been "deaf as a post," he asserted, and had regained some hearing after tank treatments. She was a sister of Henry H. Timken of Canton, Ohio, multi-millionaire head of the Timken Roller Bearing Empire.

Rand pondered this medical tidbit. He wondered if the treatments could help his wife. Rand was at the point of desperation in trying to cope with the hypertension that was wrecking his wife's life. He had taken her to clinics all over America and to a few abroad. No doctor had been able to substantially lower her blood pressure. Being an invalid was supremely galling to Miriam Smith Rand, a vivacious beauty in her 30s.

After checking up on Cunningham, Rand took his wife to Kansas City. Her blood pressure was dangerously elevated, around 200 systolic. The doctor examined her and speculated that compressed-air treatment would help her; and it did. Gradually her pressure fell to about 150. Cunningham advised the Rands this was by no means a cure, and that her pressure probably would rise again. But meantime, she could resume her normal life, and come back for more treatments in the tank in a few weeks when her blood pressure again reached dangerous levels. Thus, her way of life became a series of in-and-out visits to The Tank, but that was better than being continually ill.

Near disaster struck the sanitarium in the winter of 1923.

"The tanks on fire!"

An anguished cry over the intercom from the inside nurse brought Cunningham on the run. He couldn't believe it; patients had been warned not to smoke, every precaution taken. The doctor plunged into the entry lock, saw hazy smoke in the left compartment and quickly herded out all the patients, and then emptied the other end of the tank. There seemed to be nothing on fire, but part of the floor was charred. Nobody was hurt and damaged was minor; but Cunningham angrily investigated what had gone wrong. He was considerably chagrined. He had installed open gas burners under the tank to keep it warm in winter. Somebody had turned the flame a little too high and scorched the interior insulation. That never happened again.

By this time, there were so many patients, Cunningham had to enlarge his sanitarium. He purchased the big three-story residence next door at 3316 Harrison and built a second tank 10 by 100 feet. It was more luxurious, with one chamber furnished like a fine living room, including a piano.

Mindful of the close-call fire, he enclosed this tank inside a concrete block building to insulate it from vagaries of the weather. The building's windows were lined up with the tank's portholes so patients could easily look out onto the street.

Some patients lived in the tank for seven days, five days at full pressure of about 3 ATA, and the final two days in stage decompression, dropping five pounds every 12 hours. Both tanks were kept busy.

Financial success came. The Bagby loan was paid off. The sanitarium deposited so much money in the nearby Linwood Avenue bank that Cunningham was elected a bank director. The Cunninghams moved to a house in the country club district. His Chandler sedan was replaced by a shiny new Marmon, then a Packard—and finally two Packard sedans were in his garage. His net income had reached $100,000 a year.

His fees were $3 for the day treatment, $6 overnight. He quoted $306 per month to treat a young diabetic girl, presumably including meals. He estimated it would cost $2,600 monthly to staff and run a single-tank sanitarium which should gross $31,000 a month.

Late in 1924, he got a new patient who changed the whole course of his career, and the history of hyperbaric medicine.

The formerly deaf Mrs. Reynolds sent her brother, the Timken Bearing tycoon. Ordinarily, the fifty-six-year-old Henry H. Timken had a visage perfectly typifying the stereotype of aristocratic hauteur. But he came to the sanitarium at night, puffy and ugly from his own poison, writhing in pain, at the ragged edge of delirium.

There was not a moment to lose. The man had uremic poisoning, and Cunningham put him in the tank at once. Had the sick man waited too long? Timken, a man reputed able to write a check for one hundred twenty million dollars, was sinking fast. Through the night come the fight for life see-sawed. Cunningham stayed at his patient's side in the tank and went through one cliffhanger crisis after another. Timken frequently sank into a coma. Finally, after about sixty hours, the tycoon's fever broke, and he began to rally. After a few more days, Timken was able to emerge from the chamber and convalesce in the sanitarium building. Realist Timken saw one thing clearly—Cunningham's tank had saved his life!

He expressed boundless verbal appreciation but wanted to do more. Finally, he thought of something. He offered to build for Cunningham the biggest compressed air tank in the world—large enough to hold an entire hospital!

The doctor was stunned. He couldn't believe Timken could be serious. But he was. Timken suggested erecting the big tank in Cleveland so his engineers from the Canton works could help erect it.

"Mr. Timken, what do you have in mind—in dollar value?" Cunningham asked.

Timken said calmly, "One million dollars."

"I'd be a fool, Mr. Timken, not to leap at that."

They shook hands on it.

The page one drama that traumatized America in 1925 was the saga of spelunker Floyd Collins, trapped in a cave in Kentucky with heroic rescuers frantically digging day and night—but reaching him too late. It was to Cunningham, the most significant year of a controversial medical career, if not of his entire life. He had just turned forty-five; he and Grace now had two children, a baby daughter named Dorothy and a son, Orval, Jr., then 10 years old.

The agreement with Timken had been formalized. They were to be equal partners in the Cleveland venture. They were on the verge of acquiring a building site, and Cunningham spent hours pummeling his fertile brain for a design concept.

The Kansas City sanitarium complex in 1925 was booming. Both tanks ran almost continuously. By this time, no less than three thousand patients had been treated. Cunningham also moved his Goat Hill tank to Harrison Avenue so he and his friend, Professor Nelson, could use it for further animal experiments.

Cunningham was losing some of his high standing with the doctors in Kansas City. As an inventive, skillful anesthetist, he had been needed and wanted by surgeons. Everyone in his classes seemed to rate him an excellent teacher. But now that he was driving a Packard sedan and offering therapy that his peers did not believe had been adequately tested and proved, the climate grew increasingly cool.

Much carping poured into the ears of Dean Sudler. He defended Cunningham who continued to fully meet his campus obligations despite the busy sanitarium. In a letter to Chancellor Strong on February 14th, 1925, Dean Sudler touched on the growing feud among the faculty doctors:

"Dr Cunningham is engaged in a certain type of research work over the merits of which there is a great difference of opinion, some regarding it highly, others as pernicious."

The upshot of the dissension was that finally Sudler was required to dispatch a very formal letter informing Cunningham that his tenure as professor of anesthesiology would have to terminate because the medical school's regulations required teaching appointments to be made only to departments in which appointees specialized.

"You are, as we know, no longer specializing in anesthesia, the dean wrote, (with obvious personal distress) but giving your full attention to the problems of medicine.

However, I would be very pleased if you would accept an appointment in the department of medicine as associate professor. We would be honored to have a man of your distinction continue on our faculty."

The alternative offered by the letter saddened the usually stoic Cunningham. He enjoyed teaching, the chance to touch eager fresh minds. Yet, how could he continue now? The chairman of the Department of Medicine was, unfortunately, his arch-antagonist on Goat Hill. He dictated a letter terminating his connection with the University of Kansas School of Medicine.

Even this was not enough to appease his detractors. They were, for whatever motive, trying to bring heavier guns to bear on him. And they would succeed.

Meanwhile, famous people sang his praises because of The Tank's wonder healing. Miriam Smith Rand again found savor in life. Cunningham had no cure for her high blood pressure, but when it periodically became critically elevated, she would come and live in the tank for a few palliative weeks. Then, she would rush off for another whirl in Eastern Society.

No other physician in America, or the world at that particular time, was offering compressed-air therapy; and letters of inquiry poured in from all across the country. Cunningham gave matter-of-fact responses, explaining the facilities, his fees, and types of treatment. He never contended the compressed-air therapy was a total cure. "We have achieved some very beneficial results," was his usual phrase.

In July 1925, big trouble began. A letter asking pointed questions arrived from the Bureau of Investigation at the Chicago headquarters of the American Medical Association.

Cunningham did not see it at once. He was off on a trip—a very notable trip, as it turned out.

With a nurse to attend two-month-old Dorothy, Cunningham had motored north with Grace and Orval, Jr., to inspect the property in Cleveland that Timken had acquired as their hospital site. He found it to be a magnificent plot of thirteen acres on the shore of Lake Erie and eight miles east of downtown Cleveland, 18485 Lake Shore Boulevard.

Extremely pleased with this location, Cunningham drove to Canton to tell Timken so. He also wanted to talk personally with the chief engineer at the roller-bearing works, Alois Hauser, with whom he was cooperating on a design for the Cleveland project. Batting ideas back and forth in Hauser's office, they came up with a daring concept that startled them both.

The Cunningham family toured the east for a few weeks before motoring back to Kansas City. Cunningham's secretary, in some agitation, handed him the letter from the AMA. Its contents did not greatly surprise the doctor; he had expected to be challenged by Dr. Morris Fishbein, the aggressive and peripatetic editor of the prestigious Journal of the AMA and driving force behind its Bureau of Investigation. Cunningham had followed Fishbein's career, especially since both were graduates of Chicago's Rush Medical College, Cunningham in 1904, Fishbein eight years later. The Journal's editor was earning a reputation as a bold crusader against quacks and some of his biggest targets would be the goat gland specialist, patent medicine purveyors, and alcoholism clinics.

The letter pointed out that the AMA headquarters in Chicago had been receiving inquiries for more than five years about the "tank treatments" and wanted some solid information on which to base their response to questions from physicians. It asked Cunningham to answer these four questions:

What claims are made for the Cunningham treatment?

Has any report on this method of treatment been published in any medical journal? If so, what journal, and under what date?

Has the treatment been put on a commercial basis? In other words, has it been incorporated?

Has the tank, or the method by which the tank is operated, been patented?

The tone of the communication irritated Cunningham. But he was willing to comply. The best way to satisfy their curiosity would be face to face. He took the train to Chicago and went to AMA headquarters.

The journey was not a success.

The AMA didn't want to talk about it. Fishbein insisted on written answers to the questions. In summarizing the entire tank investigation nearly three years later, The Journal of the AMA (May 5th, 1928) recounted:

...In the early part of September of 1925, Dr. Cunningham came to A.M.A. headquarters to give, as he stated, the answers to the questions that had been put. It was explained to Dr. Cunningham that verbal explanations were unsatisfactory because of the possibility of misinterpretation or misconstruction, and the doctor was urged, therefore, to send to the journal, on his return to Kansas City, a written statement embodying the answers that he had given orally.

Back home, Cunningham told his wife bitterly that the A.M.A. wanted him to devote time to more animal experiments and also report examples of the treatments he was giving. Orval, Jr., in later years, said his father was "like a man with a bear by the tail—he couldn't let go. He felt his most important work was to help sick people get well."

Cunningham put off writing up anything for the AMA, and instead plunged in to catch up with his heavy patient load. His mind was occupied also with ideas for the proposed Cleveland Sanitarium. The months flew swiftly, and by his 46th birthday on January 30th, 1926, Cunningham had finished designing the "steel-ball hospital."

Cunningham knew what they planned to build would startle Cleveland—and the nation—and the world! There was nothing like it anywhere. Timken's remark about putting the whole hospital in the tank had started him thinking.

He and Houser decided to build a great steel sphere. It would stand as tall as a five-story building, and actually contain five different floors. Three would be taken up by a total of thirty-six double bedrooms, each with private bath. The ground floor would contain a dining room; the top floor would be given over to a huge recreation and game room, a place for patients to while away their hours under pressure. Elevators would connect all floors.

This sphere would be sixty-four feet in diameter—a monster in metal. But this elaborate invention was just part of the Cleveland sanitarium complex. At the base of the sphere would be located two large cylindrical tanks like those used in Kansas City. Each would be 16 feet in diameter, one 70 feet long, the other 35 feet. There would be one common entry lock, a tank about 10 by 20 feet, connecting the two tanks and the steel ball.

Even this was not all they would build. Cunningham's usual treatment now meant placing patients under pressure for one full week, alternating a week out for "rest," then another week under pressure, and so on. Cunningham decided to provide accommodations for his clients during the "out" period. Close by the Cleveland tanks would be erected a handsome three-story brick hotel, a rather large one. And there would be still another brick building to house the power plant, compressors, boilers, air conditioning machinery, all the works.

At Timken's insistence, all furnishings were to be luxurious, as fine as the best New York hotel. The cylindrical tanks would have plush Pullman compartments, quite roomy with comfortable berths 3 by 7 feet. To avoid fire hazards, no wood would be used anywhere inside. Daylight would enter the sphere through 350 portholes each 10 inches in diameter.

Compressors would provide 3,100 cubic feet of air per minute and the sphere would be air conditioned at 68 to 70 degrees with 65 to 68% humidity. It would be positioned to rest on rollers atop concrete piers and thus accommodate heat expansion caused by the sun shining on the metal. But it could withstand a 100-mile-an-hour gale. Cunningham estimated it would be a year before the complex could be built and in use.

Those were indeed busy days, but finally, in February, Cunningham wrote answers to the A.M.A. questions. In the eventual summary of the investigation, the Journal said of that communication:

"Dr. Cunningham sent in a reply to the questions asked seven months previously. In his answer to the first question, Dr. Cunningham said, in effect, that his method of treatment was a "practical and efficient method of administering oxygen"; that it would produce temporary beneficial results in cases of high blood pressure, acidosis, and conditions needing heart rest; that relief had been obtained in "the treatment of some anaphylactic conditions, as hay fever and asthma"; that syphilitic patients with a positive Wassermann became, after treatment, negative and that tabetic pains, when present, were quickly relieved; that the treatment apparently cured many cases of diabetes mellitus, hypertrophic arthritis and pernicious anemia. For the somewhat surprising claims, no evidence was submitted.

Dr Cunningham's answer to the second question was that he had published no clinical reports on the effects of compressed air therapy. To question three, he replied that the treatments had not been put on a commercial basis nor had it been incorporated. To question four, Dr. Cunningham stated that, while there were no patents, so far as he knew, that would prevent anyone from giving compressed air treatments, he has secured a patent on certain mechanical features which affect economics in the compression and use of compressed air."

Cunningham's response obviously was not sufficient to erase the skepticism that existed in AMA headquarters. In the interim, Dr. Nelson had partially injected himself into the controversy. He sent to Fishbein the reprint of an article that he and Parke Woodard had done on "The Relief of Experimental Arterial and Anoxemia by Compressed Air." The article appeared originally in the Journal of Pathology and Bacteriology of London. In essence, it said that normal anesthetized rabbits, when subjected to compressed air pressure, showed an increase in the arterial oxygen saturation and the carbon dioxide content. Nearly three decades later, other experimenters would demonstrate the same effect, making possible the world-famous sensational "blue-baby" surgery of the late 50s. But back in 1926, the Journal of the AMA did not appear to be impressed by Nelson's work.

Nelson's letter made one statement that must have prompted Fishbein to jot a memo on his calendar. Cunningham, according to Nelson, was about ready to report on his clinical findings, and the material would appear in the Journal of the Kansas Medical Society. That may have been projected; but what of Cunningham's old enemies on Goat Hill, and other envious local doctors? Do they have any influence over whose articles saw the light of print in the

Kansas Medical Society's publication? The answer seems obvious, considering another excerpt from the Bureau of Investigations final report in the Journal of the AMA:

Dr. Cunningham was again written to in July 1926 and asked (because of what Nelson had said) if he had published any report. The letter was ignored—at least, no answer has ever been received.

In the April 1927 issue of a small publication known as Anesthesia and Analgesia there appeared under the title "Oxygen Therapy by Means of Compressed Air" what is, apparently, the first and only printed statement by Dr. Cunningham regarding his work. The article was stated to have been read before the Mid-Western Association of Anesthetists, which met in Kansas City in October 1926.

From this article, and from a great many letters on file written to laymen by Dr. Cunningham, it appears that the doctor's thesis is that diabetes mellitus, hypertrophic arthritis and carcinoma are all due to the bacteria of the anaerobic type. He holds further that the oxygen content of the tissues is greatly increased when the patients are put in his compressed air tank and that the compressed air treatment is curative in certain cases of diabetes mellitus, pernicious anemia, hypertrophic arthritis, syphilis, and carcinoma...

Another year was allowed to elapse, and in June 1927, Dr. Cunningham was again asked for a report that would make possible the checking up of the results claim for the tank treatment. He stated in reply to this request that he was preparing such a report. As nothing further was heard from the doctor, he was again written to two months later—September 7th, 1927. Dr. Cunningham stated that he had been away most of the summer on a vacation trip but would "begin at once gathering data and making check-ups on patients for the report, which I shall be able to submit to you in 60 days." This was more than seven months ago, and the report has not been received.

It became increasingly clear to Fishbein that Cunningham, for whatever reason, was unwilling or unable to supply the kind of prompt and thorough scientific accounting the powerful American Medical Association thought it had the right to expect from medical experimenters or clinical entrepreneurs. The editor of the Journal of the AMA then began loading his devastating artillery for the direct bombardment he was to turn loose within a few months on Cunningham.

At this point, Miriam Rand was again in the Kansas City sanitarium. Her husband, pleased with what Cunningham had managed to do for her, was off pursuing one of his hobbies—speedboat racing. He was in Detroit to run a highly unorthodox race.

It was his speed boat against the Ford Trimotor passenger plane. This was the year of the birth of part-talkies; The Jazz Singer was wowing 'em at the Roxy in New York. The nation had gone airplane crazy. In May, Lindberg had stunningly soloed the Atlantic, 3,610 miles to Paris in 33 ½ hours.

Rand may have suspected a public relations gimmick in the water-sky race on the Detroit River. He beat the airplane. But Henry Ford, handing him the trophy, had a one-two punch; he talked Rand into taking a ride in the Trimotor.

Henry Ford was a super-salesman. In the air, Rand became so impressed that he bought the Trimotor. He promptly engaged a pilot and a co-pilot and set out for Kansas City. He could hardly wait to show Miriam her new present.

Mrs. Rand was elated. The site of the gleaming airplane sent her spirits into the clouds, and she wanted to fly at once to New York. Cunningham briskly shook his head and cautioned that she had been getting better in the tank because of living under maximum low-altitude conditions. On this plane, she would be in high altitude, in rarefied air. Just the opposite of what had helped her.

Miriam Rand looked at her doctor, frowning. At length, she gave an eloquent shrug. She reached for her husband's hand. "Doctor, I'm sorry. I've just got to fly now!"

The Trimotor streaked off into the afternoon sky. All went well until the aircraft ran head-on into a heavy thunderstorm over northern Ohio and made an emergency landing at Lima, Ohio. The Rands summoned a taxi, and by night were speeding east aboard the Twentieth Century Limited. Miriam Rand was gay. In the club car she had a grand slam in no trump and made it. Elated, she said good night and went down the corridor to their compartment. Rand heard a heavy thud and ran to the compartment. Miriam Rand lay slumped in her doorway. She had suffered a stroke. An ambulance and doctor met the train in Rochester, but she was already dead.

This tragedy triggered two decisions by Rand that were markedly to influence the conclusion of the saga of the Kansas City compressed-air doctor. Fourteen-year-old James H. Rand III turned very restless after his mother's death. So, Cunningham took him on as an adolescent protégé in the lab. And the boy became an HBO expert.

The experience inspired him on to become a famous research scientist, noted now for a host of inventions. Among them, the metal cloth milium. Also come the first electric massager-shock device that overcomes cardiac arrest. He developed a pressure-point mattress for hospitals to banish bed sores, a famous washing machine, an electric shaver, seatless water valves, and many more. In World War II, he was the gutsy ramrod of the U.S. guided missile attack against the Nazis. He became Cleveland's 1949 Man of the Year. He later developed a disputed "cancer vaccine" which the U. S. Food and Drug Administration outlawed a few years ago—but on which he began further testing in Mexico.

In those Kansas City days, destiny also was grooming Jimmy Rand for a starring role in the drama of the steel-ball hospital in Cleveland.

The other notable decision by the elder Rand was to try to interest his alma mater, Harvard University, in compressed air medical experimentation, as a tribute to his wife. He offered to have a tank built for the School of Public Health and wrote out a check for $100,000 establishing the Miriam Smith Rand Fund.

Meanwhile, construction was starting in Cleveland. The Biggs Boiler Works Company of Akron, Ohio, got the contract to fabricate—no small undertaking—the steel ball, plus the other tanks. Melbourne Construction Company of Canton, Ohio, was employed as general contractor.

In the beginning, a high wall was thrown up around the property on Lakeshore Boulevard. Guards were posted and no outsiders were admitted. There was an air of total secrecy. Timken had always been publicity-shy; but this conduct was much more mysterious than Cunningham had ever before displayed.

The Cleveland newspapers were curious, and reporters kept pecking away until they were finally able to break the news early in 1928 that Timken was erecting the "steel ball" sanitarium to treat principally diabetes. Cunningham refused to talk to any reporters, explaining "I do not wish accounts to describe the treatment and the tank as foolish."

The secrecy surrounding the work in Cleveland kept bringing a flurry of questions, ridicule, and denunciation. An editorial in The Plain Dealer contrasted Timken's secrecy with the openness with which Cleveland philanthropist Samuel Mather had given $5,000,000 to the Western Reserve University Medical Center. Timken's sanitarium, said the newspaper, would be under suspicion by the entire medical profession until it came out from behind the fence.

Two spokesmen for the Cleveland Academy of Medicine echoed the criticism and went even further. Dr. J. F. Tuckerman and Dr. A. B. Denison were quoted in the Cleveland Press:

1. That they had never seen in print within the last five years any description by Dr Cunningham of his system.
2. That in keeping details of a system secret, he made it impossible for other medical experimenters to test his system.
3. That there is no proof that diabetes or any of the other diseases, which it is understood the sanitarium will treat, are caused by anaerobic germs.
4. That oxygen in the bloodstream is carried by the hemoglobin, the coloring matter in the red corpuscles of the blood, and that experiments have shown it is saturated with oxygen at ordinary air pressure. This means that no more oxygen could be introduced into it by increased pressure since it already holds as much as it can.
5. That experiments have shown that increased air pressure introduced an infinitesimal amount of the extra oxygen in the blood serum but that no one has ever shown that this does any good or will, in any way affect the course of any disease.

Cunningham ignored his critics. But the attacks stung. To Grace, he appeared "just terribly crushed" when the AMA finally published its lengthy Bureau of Investigation account in the Journal in May 1928, concluding:

...(Dr. Cunningham) has published no case reports or furnished the medical profession with any evidence to support the claims. Under the circumstances, is it to be wondered at if the medical profession looks askance at the "tank treatment" and intimates that it seems tinctured much more strongly with economics than with scientific medicine? It is a mark of the scientist that he is ready to make available the evidence on which his claims are based. Dr. Cunningham has been given repeated opportunities to present such evidence.

This was the dark hour before a bright dawn. Despite the mountain of doubts and the flood of derision, the "Timken Tank" or "steel-ball hospital" was finally completed in December 1928. Reporters at last were given a tour of inspection. They were genuinely impressed—and why not? The complex would be a marvel even today!

Cunningham shut down his Kansas City tanks, and the compressed-air boom promptly exploded in Cleveland. The Cleveland Academy of Medicine rejected his application for membership. But that certainly didn't keep patients away. Famous people from all across the nation continue to flock to Cunningham. The wealthy found his new tanks and hotel fitted with costly oriental rugs and lush drapes equal to theirs at home.

In the steel ball's fifth floor card room, Frank Sieberling, the Akron tire tycoon, might be found at 3 ATA puffing a cigarette and playing for high poker stakes while in the dining salon below, a delectable lunch was served by attendants to a member of Philadelphia's Shibe baseball clan.

Once an ash dropped from a cigarette on Seiberling's tweed jacket and flared up. It was no real cause for alarm. Anticipating the hazard, Cunningham had installed automatic showers. Someone just shoved Seiberling under the sprinkler.

As business boomed, Cunningham added to his staff of technicians and nurses, occupied a mansion on the grounds, bought a Cadillac and a lake cruiser, sent his son to an exclusive prep school—and finally found enough leisure for some further experimental work.

He wanted to really pit the tank against cancer. One of the Shibes put up $20,000 to finance the experiment. From New York's Welfare Island, twenty-two men with terminal cancer were brought to the Cleveland sanitarium.

Young Jimmy Rand, who happened to be "free" while transferring from the University of Virginia to the University of Vienna, helped give these patients their treatments. "They died like flies," Rand recalled in a 1972 interview. "Three or four didn't; they probably had spontaneous remissions. You must remember that these were all terminal. I went into the tank one morning and found one poor devil had hanged himself. All of them must have figured they were goners—maybe Cunningham could do something for them. But nothing ever came of it."

Cunningham also speculated, Rand recalled, that negative pressure, a partial vacuum, would lessen withdrawal symptoms of narcotic addicts. He had heard that because mile-high Denver has a rarefied atmosphere, addicts there could practically quit cold turkey without ill effects in his garage, Cunningham built a small tank in which pressure could be reduced to one-half atmosphere, or about seven pounds per square inch. Rand helped Cunningham confine two drug users in this tank for five days. "He was right as rain," Rand recalls, "sure enough, no withdrawal symptoms."

To prove his point, Cunningham put two men who had gone back on dope into the tank. Rand said he just locked the door, made no pressure change at all, just sea level atmosphere. "Those guys went through hell," Rand says, "ripped their clothes, vomited—it was awful. But it was a worthwhile experiment. I tried to find the records on it. Like so many others, they are lost."

Cunningham could withstand the tough opposition of medical fraternity leaders, but he was no match for a nationwide economic collapse. Just as the stock market crashed and the 1929 Depression hit, Timken soured on the steel ball hospital, too. It is not entirely clear why; his heirs who still control the roller-bearing empire brush aside all inquiries with polite vagueness. Cunningham's heirs don't have an explanation either.

The bubble spawned back on Goat Hill during the World War I flu epidemic was about to burst—and there was no stopping it.

With money suddenly scarce, business fell off drastically, under the imminent threat of Timken's withdrawal, Cunningham felt his whole life tottering. It literally was. He had developed serious heart trouble. Ironically, he didn't seek benefits for his own health in the tank; he didn't think it would help his condition.

Where would he find somebody to rescue the steel-ball hospital? Finally, he thought of Jimmy Rand, his young protégé who was just about to turn 21 years old, and who had a wealthy father who knew first-hand the value of the compressed-air marvel.

Young Jimmy was willing. His father was not. For one thing, Rand senior was financially in deep water himself, along with thousands of other floundering, once-mighty industrialists.

Timken insisted on a settlement. Young Jimmy made an offer—a down payment of 30-thousand dollars inherited from his mother, provided he could have a year to raise the balance of the $500,000 asking price.

On September 28th, 1934, it was announced that James H. Rand III of New York City, a "research marvel" and son of the Remington-Rand president, had bought the Cleveland sanitarium for half a million dollars.

The ailing Cunningham wished the new owner good luck, moved off the grounds, and found another house in Cleveland. Young Rand promptly teamed up with a red-faced, fast-talking real estate promoter named Applegate. The promoter happened to be the boyfriend of Cunningham's former secretary.

The name of the sanitarium was promptly changed to Ohio Institute of Oxygen Therapy. Young Rand hired a couple of doctors from Columbus through a want ad. But the medical watchdogs who had been after Cunningham's scalp slashed even more viciously at the new owner. From the start, the "research marvel" was doomed, and he was too innocent to know it.

The magic was gone. No patients came—none.

Even ten dollars or so a day might have kept the place in business. Applegate flitted about Ohio, trying to pedal stock in the institute. It was tough going. Rand tried to lease out the sanitarium, or part of it. Could it be turned into a tuberculosis hospital? Or a mental institution?

Some complaints were made about Applegate's stock deals. The Ohio Attorney General took a dim view and started a "blue sky law" investigation that added to the troubles of the harried young owner.

But Jimmy Rand refused to surrender. He remembered a vice-president at IBM, a former Cunningham patient. He rushed to New York to appeal to him, but in vain. He then thought the government should take over the sanitarium as a research center. Rand went to Washington and got an appointment with the Surgeon General. He managed to spark some interest; and that hung fire for several weeks. Then it fizzled.

The one year of time that Jimmy Rand's thirty grand had bought came to an end. He asked Timken for more time. But the roller-bearing tycoon wanted everything over and done. He took back the sanitarium. The steel ball and the tanks were shut down; the giant power plant was darkened; the hotel was shuttered. Later Timken gave it all to the Catholic Youth Organization.

The turn of events saddened Cunningham, who now had painful congestive heart failure. He knew his days were numbered, but he attempted one more invention. He had an idea for a sprocketless movie projector. This would make it possible to bring the best teachers in the world on film into the poorest of classrooms. Once again, he was ahead of his time. But soon his heart became so crippled that he had to stop work altogether. On February 23rd, 1937, not quite a month after his 57th birthday, he died.

Perhaps fate, after all, was kind to Orval Cunningham. He was spared witnessing the ignominious end of his Cleveland dream. To salvage a paltry $25,000 worth of steel for the World War II effort, the U.S. War Production Board on March 31st, 1942, ordered wreckers to completely dismantle the million-dollar steel ball hospital, the like of which the world never saw before—or since!

5

"OPEN" SECRET AT HARVARD

Dr. William F. Bernhard, brilliant young cardiovascular surgeon at Children's Medical Center in Boston, was anxious to duplicate the "blue baby" hyperbaric surgery he just learned was performed in Amsterdam.

He needed the kind of surgical pressure tank the Dutch had built—and he didn't know of anything like that in the United States.

Perhaps he could get by using a Navy decompression chamber. He went to the Commandant of the submarine medical school at New London, Connecticut.

Bernhardt's request stunned the Navy officer. "Don't you know, Doctor, there is a marvelous hyperbaric chamber just a hundred feet behind your hospital!"

Bernhardt did not, in fact, know that the Harvard School of Public Health had the epochal Miriam Smith Rand hyperbaric chamber tucked into a concrete block annex at the rear of their 55 Shattuck Street main building. In 1962, it had been there thirty-four years, quietly spawning medical history milestones, a sort of "open" secret at Harvard Med. Bernhard can be excused his ignorance; even today, many people at work on the Harvard campus still don't know that the tank is there.

The American Medical Association has never uttered a critical word about this tank, although it was directly inspired by Dr. Cunningham's Goat Hill experiments. It is his indirect legacy to every hyperbaric researcher who followed, and stoutly ties his long shadow from the controversial past directly to current developments in the field.

Except for his complete faith and confidence in Cunningham results, Miriam Rand's husband would not have pressed this tank on his alma mater. The Biggs Boiler Works Co. of Akron built the tank for Harvard at the same time it was fabricating the marvelous steel-ball hospital for Cleveland. Harvard's tank was delivered to Boston in 1928 at the same time the Cleveland sanitarium was opening. In essence, Cunningham's fingerprints were all over the Harvard tank. But it never suffered from the taint that haunted his own pressure chambers.

Had an alumnus of lesser stature or influence offered the gift, Harvard surely would have declined. Dr. Cecil K. Drinker, dean of the School of Public Health, managed only minimal enthusiasm at that. Rand was convinced there was something big here—potential medical breakthrough discoveries. What he sought was a vigorous broad-range inquiry into all aspects of clinical therapeutic pressurization.

"But they never did it," his son, James H. Rand III, told me in 1972. "They went into oxygen poisoning. Hell, they proved what was already known. Drinker wasn't really interested, and he did have to start from scratch in this. My father thought Harvard was dragging its feet. They never really did anything."

It is true that the tank was largely ignored in years that could have been devoted to profitable experimentation. Belatedly, it did get fairly heavy and serious use. It became the scene of a variety of notable triumphs—and one grim failure, before the eyes of the nation, the loss of a famous patient in a dramatic and risky eleventh-hour gamble.

The tank—eight feet in diameter and thirty-one feet long, divided into two separate chambers by a central entry lock—was installed in November 1928. It was the first device of its kind on any American campus (except for the much cruder tank on Goat

Hill). The Harvard tank costs Rand $30,000—and would run about $200,000 if duplicated today.

Constantin P. Yaglou, professor of industrial hygiene, designed it; he later became an international authority on human adaptation to climate extremes.

But about all the professors at Harvard seemed to want to do initially was just stroll by and look at the iron monster. It was a nifty tank. Not only hyperbaric, but also hypobaric. Yaglou engineered it to achieve 60 pounds per square inch absolute pressure (above 6 ATA), or to reduce pressure down to about six pounds per square inch (slightly less than one half ATA).

Even today's sophisticated and improved communication methods leave us frequently unaware of timely events that critically affect our lives; but it was obviously worse in those days—at the close of the 1920s. The right hand of science never seemed to be quite up on where the left was tinkering.

Somehow in 1932, the Navy got wind of the Harvard tank. Diving studies had been going on at the Brooklyn Navy Yard since 1915, but the Navy thought this new chamber looked like a valuable tool and they'd like to experiment with it.

Harvard was willing. A young Navy doctor, Albert H. Behnke, took charge. The big worry was how much oxygen man could tolerate under pressure, and for how long. British scientists had been daring the depths for twenty-five years. One, John Scott Haldane, reported amnesia on diving to 300 feet. And G.C.C. Damant and A.E. Phillips had convulsed at 4 ATA. Behnke began two years of human experiments and proved that Haldane's amnesia was caused by nitrogen bubbling in his blood and unable to escape. Behnke became a research great and eventually retired as an Admiral.

By the early thirties, when the Cleveland steel-ball hospital was forced to close, world interest and hyperbaric medicine was down to about zero. An exception was Milwaukee. There, the fresh young mind of Dr. Edgar End was at large in the caisson workers' emergency tank. A diver, Max Nohl, teamed up with him and they began testing gas mixtures. Nohl wanted to set a diving record. They hit on a helium-oxygen mixture; and on December 1st, 1937, Nohl at age 27 dropped into frigid Lake Michigan and sank to 420 feet to set a new world record. This was more than just daredevilry; it was pushing back medical frontiers. End, then also 27, went on to important hyperbaric discoveries that rank him as a top authority.

Major research emphasis was on diving problems. This single-mindedness apparently kept everybody from seeing the potential right under their noses when in 1939, Dr. Robert Gross, chief surgeon at the Boston Children's Medical Center, did his first corrective heart surgery on a blue baby. Yet his scalpel flashed under operating lights that were barely 100 feet from the Harvard tank. The possibility of doing hyperbaric blue-baby operations hadn't been thought of yet. And Bill Bernhard was only a 14-year-old kid playing kick-the-can on a Brooklyn Street. Twenty-three years were to roll by before Bernhard would be doing America's first hyperbaric surgery in the Harvard tank.

"The Squalus has sunk! Three hundred feet down! We've got to find a gas mixture that will let us go that deep and save the crew. May we use your tank again?"

Harvard heard that distress cry from Behnke in June 1939. The submarine had gone down off Portsmouth, New Hampshire. The crew of 59 was trapped. Behnke and C. B. (Swede) Momson worked frantically in the Harvard tank. They tried one experiment after another until they hit on the right calculation. Their fresh knowledge was what the bell rescuers needed, and thirty-three men were brought up from the sub alive.

Then in 1940, the dark clouds of World War II gathered.

Even in retrospect, it is difficult to be charitable about Washington's bureaucratic blunder in ordering destruction of the steel-ball hospital. On the very day this death knell was being typed out, the Air Force was urgently seeking a pressure chamber in which to develop suitable oxygen masks for the US bomber crews to wear at high altitude.

The Air Force took over the smaller and less suitable Harvard tank; and running the oxygen mask experiments kept it humming for five years. From that work also came an improved microphone for high altitude communication. And much later, in 1952, the tank was used as a "shock tube" in designing non-contaminant filters for the Atomic Energy Commission.

Then once more, interest abruptly died. The Harvard tank was dark except once a year when it was pressurized to give industrial hygiene students an orientation dive, a tiny taste of the caisson worker environment. There were some other impromptu uses. Harvard's rowing teams sat inside daily at hypobaric pressure for a couple weeks to get used to the feel of mile-high altitude before going to the Mexico City Olympics. A couple of Harvard professors used the tank for small research projects. Dr. Guido Majno pressurized small animals seeking a new explanation for the bends. Dr. Jere Mead measured inert gases in the lungs.

The Europeans discovered oxygen and why it is necessary for life; they invented air compressors, diving suits, submarines, and the caisson system. They also were far ahead of American scientists in trying to effectively utilize hyperoxygenation, though perhaps their le bain d'air comprime episodes had best be forgotten. So, it is not at all surprising that in the early 1950s, the Europeans suddenly again got all steamed up about hyperbaric medicine.

The new interest erupted in several cities practically simultaneously—in London, in Glasgow, in Amsterdam.

British doctors, starting in 1954, were the first. They began using hyperbaric pressure in connection with radiation of cancer patients. Dr. Ian Churchill-Davidson reported surprisingly good results at St.

Thomas' Hospital in London. Of course, this led to experiments with other diseases.

In Scotland, doctors at Glasgow's Western Infirmary pirated the hospitals discarded autoclave. They converted it—reminiscent of Goat Hill thirty-eight years earlier—into a chamber at modest cost. It was good enough for animal experiments, and these looked very promising.

Then in Amsterdam, along came husky, energetic Professor Ite Boerema—now known as "the father of hyperbaric medicine." He wanted to use a chamber for surgery, especially on blue babies.

As Boerema explains it, the normal human body is like a sponge soaked with oxygen. Diseases will dry out the sponge, as does injury, a faulty heart, crippled lungs. He reasoned that pressure will drive oxygen back in.

Boerema had no chamber and no experience in one. An hour's drive from Wilhelmina Hospital, he found a Royal Dutch Navy decompression chamber and borrowed its use. He rigged it up as a crude operating room. Then he went in, dogged the door, turned up the pressure and practiced on animals to test his theory that a body could be literally drenched with oxygen.

His prize patient was a pig. Boerema bled out all the animal's red blood cells—under triple atmospheric pressure—and replaced the healthy whole blood with colorless synthetic plasma. Normally, such a procedure would bring death within four minutes. But this pig in the tank lived. For 90 minutes, the animal did just fine—except for turning white. The quantity of his bodily oxygen had increased 10 times normal. Boerema could see his pig literally was drenched, and the plasma alone was carrying all the oxygen. (Which the Cleveland Academy of Medicine spokesman in rebuking Cunningham had unwisely said could not be done.)

Boerema was walking on air; now he had a way of protecting blue babies while he operated on their frail hearts. With true Dutch thrift, he is said to have sold the pig, none the worse for making medical history after its whole blood was restored, back to the farmer from whom he had bought it.

The elated Boerema readily shared his findings with other European physicians in 1956 meetings at Stockholm and Zurich. These doctors listened with interest, and promptly put the whole business out of their minds. On the strength of what he had done with the pig, however, Boerema was able to talk his hospital into building a hyperbaric operating room.

It was finished in 1959, and his first patient came in as an emergency case before he was really ready. A young girl had been waylaid, battered unconscious and abandoned for hours in a deserted field. When brought in by ambulance, she already had gas gangrene. Somebody thought to call Boerema.

The Dutch surgeon probably was not aware that as early as 1918, Cunningham had contended that oxygen under pressure would cure the anaerobic infection that causes gas gangrene. But Boerema on his own had figured that out, too. Immediately, he put the girl in his brand-new tank, his very first patient, and pulled her through.

The Glasgow doctors, meantime, got a grant of ten thousand pounds from their Health Council to build a larger chamber, a 12 by 18-foot tank that was put in use in June 1960.

Boerema kept his tank busy. All across Holland, doctors were impressed by the "miracle" of his initial gas-gangrene triumph. Within weeks, similar cases were being rushed to the tank. And Boerema also moved finally into his blue-baby surgery.

But not before he wrote two articles that were destined to trigger the modern rebirth of HBO in America. One was a technical description of his hyperbaric operating room. The other with Drs. W.H. Brummelkamp and J. Hogendijk as co-authors related the gas-gangrene miracle, explaining treatment of anaerobic infections by HBO "drenching."

Both appeared in the March 1961 issue of Surgery, the prestigious medical journal that reaches 10,000 physicians in the United States.

Boerema's success stirred imaginations all across the country. But nothing was done immediately, for every physician interested in attempting to duplicate the Dutchman's extraordinary achievements shared a common obstacle. Nobody had a hyperbaric tank.

Some doctors were aggressive enough to begin trying to overcome this shortcoming—in Chicago, Minneapolis, Durham, N.C., Baltimore, Milwaukee, Detroit, Boston...

The surgical mind that became inflamed in Boston belonged to Bernhard, who by that year had become an associate in surgery on the Harvard faculty and at Children's Medical Center was the promising protégé of Dr. Gross, the pioneer in blue-baby surgery.

So, in 1962, Bernhard went three hundred miles to New London, Connecticut to discover the Harvard tank just outside his window.

At his urging, Children's Medical Center got use of the tank on a dollar-a-year lease. Bernhard set about enthusiastically collecting the men and materials he would need to convert the tank into an operating room. He was eager to get started. He couldn't believe his good fortune; he had a hyperbaric chamber that would accommodate a surgical team, and he didn't know of any other surgeon in America who had such a facility.

But other medical experimenters were also aggressive—and imaginative. One such was Dr Alan P. Thal at Wayne State University School of Medicine in Detroit. He believed HBO would help a young {black} man he was treating for sickle-cell crisis. He had a small tank, two by four feet, for animal experiments; but that was too small to accommodate his patient. He had a sudden brainstorm—why not use a submarine?

Thal did a lot of wrangling and pleading. And finally, the Navy tied up a training sub at the docks on the Detroit River.

"It was quite an experience," Thal recalls. "First, we couldn't take the patient aboard in his stretcher. There's only one way to get aboard a sub, straight down the ladder. So, we lowered him by sling. Then we just closed up all the hatches and pressurized the hull to two atmospheres. We didn't move, didn't submerge, just stayed at the dock. The Detroit harbor is no place for a submarine to try to cruise about on the bottom."

The sub remained buttoned up for two hours. The sick man got much better—a result now uniformly achieved in sickle-cell crises by HBO clinicians. Thal had envisioned extensive use of the Navy's submarines in hyperbaric medicine. An excellent thought: but his struggle to borrow just one for a single treatment was so disillusioning, he did not long pursue human experiments in the field.

At the beginning of 1962, what amounted to an unofficial race was on between a handful of energetic physicians to get something substantial started. All had been inspired by the articles in Surgery.

Dr. Ivan W. Brown, Jr., at Duke University Medical Center, Durham, N.C., had become so caught up in this new idea that he twice flew to Amsterdam in 1961 to see Boerema and observe his drenching techniques.

For about $10,000, Brown had obtained a fully instrumented animal experiment unit: two stacked steel chambers, each not quite as large as a barrel. In these, he began testing blood-oxygen levels in dogs.

Brown told his Duke colleagues they ought to consider a larger chamber, perhaps eight by twenty feet, roomy enough for surgery on human beings.

One of Brown's friendly Rivals was Dr R. Adams Cowley, professor of surgery at University of Maryland School of Medicine at Baltimore. Though his department was short of funds, Cowley saw HBO as a possible gateway through which his personal crusade against shock trauma could advance. It literally horrified this innovative and tireless surgeon that 316 Americans are still dying daily from accidents. Cowley is unable to write off these fatalities as merely unfortunate, inevitable—something that only happens to "the other guy."

He wanted a tool that would enable emergency room surgeons to overcome the shock brought on in these accidents by sudden and heavy blood loss. The hyperbaric chamber might just turn the trick. Cowley intended to find out—and he wouldn't let an empty purse thwart him.

He salvaged an old autoclave just seventeen inches in diameter by forty-eight inches long, normally a steam pressure cooker for sterilizing surgical instruments. He jerry-rigged it into a hyperbaric chamber, piping oxygen out of standard 2,000 pounds to the square inch compressed gas cylinder. Thus, he was able to bring his little test chamber up to 3 ATA.

Then Cowley and his colleagues set out to see what HBO's effect would be against hemorrhagic shock. As a test, they produced vascular collapse in 30 dogs by bleeding out most of their blood, leaving them in critical condition for two and a half hours. Then Cowley's team went to work and used the best of conventional anti-shock techniques, but 83% of these dogs died.

Nineteen dogs were then bled in a similar fashion and after two and a half hours were treated with oxygen under three atmospheres absolute. Only 26 per cent of them died.

Cowley, reporting these experiments before the American Association of Thoracic Surgery at St Louis, April 16th-18, 1962, credited his little homemade tank with this improvement in survival rates. Indeed, it had made the difference. But then in the floor discussion on the paper, Duke's Brown sadly observed that Cowley had been playing around with a live bomb.

"I fear we did not have the courage of the Maryland group to revise one of our autoclaves for this purpose," Brown said. "I would warn that if one is going to do this, it might be worthwhile to check on the insurance carried on his laboratory and perhaps on his own life insurance to make sure he has enough, because such a pressure chamber, particularly when charged with oxygen, unless properly designed and rigidly tested, could result in a lethal accident."

Cowley shrugged off the criticism; he was already racking his brain for some scheme to get a safe chamber big enough for human experiments.

And out in Milwaukee, Dr. Carl Zenz's eyes lit up when he read the Surgery articles. For years he had been making an intensive study of man at work. St. Luke's Hospital had given him a 10 by 10 room in the basement for experimental work. Dr. Walter Thiede, a pulmonary physiology specialist, worked with him.

Luke's provided funds for a treadmill Zenz built in his own basement. Zenz obtained two small research grants and developed some interesting data. But the Amsterdam developments reminded him that he needed a sophisticated chamber in which he could simulate a great variety of environmental conditions for research. Zenz was particularly interested in the effects on workers' lungs of vanadium dust, which is increasingly used as a catalyst in industry. Thiede wanted to investigate heart and lung effects on older people who travel to high altitude. Occasionally they became acutely ill.

Zenz asked the National Institutes of Health in Washington for an $18,000 grant. Nothing doing. He tried to get $15,000 from Marquette Medical School where he was on the faculty. Another rebuff. But fortunately, he also was a medical director of the big Allis-Chalmers manufacturing works.

The officials there listened and agreed to help. Zens set about designing a 9 by 26-foot cylindrical hyperbaric chamber that would contain two locks, plus sophisticated "extras"— a treadmill and the capability of creating a 40-mile an hour wind and the temperatures from 10 below zero to 130 degrees.

This would be, of course, actually Milwaukee's second hyperbaric tank, but the design was vastly more sophisticated and modern than the old decompression unit End still had in use in County Emergency Hospital.

Zenz located a couple of special hemispherical end plates, turned over $1,400 he had left in his research coffers and hoped Allis-Chalmers could come up with a nifty tank.

About 400 miles to the Northwest, surgeons in Minneapolis also had been set buzzing by that issue of Surgery. Easily the most fascinated was Dr. Claude R. Hitchcock, chief of surgery at Minneapolis General Hospital and professor of surgery at the University of Minnesota.

He decided he absolutely must have a chamber—a big one with plenty of room for surgery. He talked it over with Dr. John J. Haglin, the hospital's assistant surgery chief, and two other surgeons, Drs. Russell H. Harris and Frank E. Johnson. They decided to make a stab at getting a tank.

Hitchcock poured over all the literature he could lay hands on. One morning, he flashed a rough penciled sketch triumphantly before his colleagues. It showed a big circular operating room with two cylindrical tanks extending from two opposite sides. Including everything, this HBO complex would cost half a million dollars, and so far, no one was prepared to put up the money.

This yearning of the Minneapolis surgeons needed no reinforcement, but they got unexpected encouragement anyhow. They were in route to Kenya to experiment on lung transplants with baboons and stopped off in Amsterdam. By this time, Boerema was used to eager and inquisitive imitators from America, and he graciously shared his knowledge with these doctors. And gave them an actual dive to demonstrate the feel of HBO.

This experience fired up Hitchcock even more. He probably decided to ask the U.S. government to finance his chamber with health research money. First, he tried to get the Congress on his side; and on March 7th, 1962, testified before the health subcommittee of the House Appropriations Committee. It was urgent, he told the congressman for America to investigate the potential of HBO, and presented a series of sketches explaining just how the body can be supersaturated with oxygen. Hitchcock predicted that eight to ten medical centers would build chambers within two years at a total cost of 10 million dollars and recommended substantial government support for this vital research. Representative Winfield K. Denton of Indiana, who presided, thanked him for appearing and observed, "That is one of the most interesting presentations we have ever had."

A few days later, Hitchcock applied to the National Institutes of Health for a quarter-million-dollar grant. His request nominated a long list of research projects. For immediate study, he proposed—as he had specifically outlined also to the Congressional subcommittee—this top priority list: 1. Carbon monoxide poisoning; 2. Anaerobic infections—gas gangrene and tetanus; 3. Severe barbiturate poisoning; 4. Severely traumatized extremities (such as compound fractures); and 5. Severe drug-induced arterial spasm. He also had a nine-point second category of "applications where research is expected to be highly productive" and a list of eight diseases nominated for "remote (Crystal Ball) Studies."

Two hospitals on the outskirts of Chicago, meanwhile, were also in this race. The effort at the new 316-bed Lutheran General Hospital in Park Ridge, Illinois, near O'Hare Airport on the north edge of the city, was sparked by Dr. Jack Van Elk, a cardiologist and Dr. Otto H. Trippel, a vascular surgeon.

Thirty-five miles to the south, in Chicago Heights, another cardiologist-surgeon team, Drs. Luke R. Pascale and Richard Wallyn, schemed to get a hyperbaric tank for use at St. James Hospital.

Since all these efforts were triggered by Boerema's articles, everybody was getting into high gear at almost the same moment. Of the lot, Van Elk was dreaming the biggest dream. He was, incidentally, a fellow countryman of Boerema's, and had come to the United States in 1954. What he envisioned for Park Ridge was the biggest hyperbaric complex in the world.

He proposed three tanks, a 10 by 41.5-foot medical chamber that would accommodate six patients on beds; a 12 by 34.5-foot surgical chamber, large enough for two operating tables and two complete surgical teams; and a 10 by 23.5-foot recompression chamber. These would lie side by side, all interconnected by lateral locks so that a person could move freely from tank to tank without being depressurized.

One million dollars was the cost estimate! That figure stunned the hospital board, but somebody recalled that the John A. Hartford Foundation of New York, established to commemorate the founder of the A & P grocery chain, was annually dispensing about 15 million dollars to 20 million dollars for medical research. Why not try them?

Van Elk was agreeable, but also impatient to get going. He had some theories on carotid- artery occlusion—a principal cause of stroke in humans—that he could test on dogs under HBO. At his urging, the hospital immediately bought an excellent small chamber for research on animals, a steel cylinder 20 by 54 inches, at a cost of $3,000.

Van Elk and Trippel began experimenting. "It was a nice chamber," Van Elk recalls, "but such small chambers have the disadvantage that the investigator cannot be inside the tank and that handling of the animal, turning stopcocks, and collecting data is difficult; however, with some ingenuity, most parameters can be measured." Then Van Elk's ingenuity created a complicated but effective hydraulic control mechanism.

The Lutheran General doctors were so encouraged by their animal tests that they decided to attempt to use the research chamber on humans—blue babies.

"We used it on three babies," Van Elk recalls "We oxygenated two babies and then took them to surgery. They did well. There was one newborn infant with a septal defect (hole in the wall between chambers in the heart) which we simply treated in the chamber, once or twice a day."

"You mean to buy time?" I asked.

"Yes. To keep the baby alive. Later it had successful surgery in a normal operating room."

It remained for this undeclared but spirited race inspired by Boerema's to be won by the other Chicago area hospital, little St. James. It was the first to acquire in response to the Amsterdam "miracles" a human chamber and treat a patient. How Pascale and Wallyn pulled this off is a dramatic and most unlikely story.

The whole problem of oxygen dissolution in the blood had intrigued Pascale for years and the news of Boerema's work, "hit me like a hammer," he says. He went to the Vacudyne Co. in Chicago Heights, a major fabricator of hyperbaric chambers.

He asked what it would take to buy one. They said about $75,000 to $100,000 for what he had in mind. The hospital didn't have that kind of budget, and he'd have to look elsewhere.

He and Wallyn had friends in the tunnel-constructing business and through them talked to the S.A. Healy Co. of Chicago. They asked to use one of Healy's decompression tanks, but because of legal implications, immediate approval wasn't given.

The very day Pascale was trying to put the bite on S. A. Healy, Jr.—May 24th, 1962—two historic events were taking place. In the space race, Navy Commander Scott Carpenter was aloft in the Mercury capsule Aurora 7, making America's first triple orbit of the earth, a year behind Russia's cosmonauts. And on the same windy day, a farmer at Lansing, Illinois, was prosaically planting evergreens, with no idea he was about to become a principal figure in the history of hyperbaric medicine.

When this man, Ralph Douma, 73, a small, wiry native of Holland, started into his house, the wind banged the door, knocking him down and driving a splinter into his hand. Douma couldn't get the splinter out but daubed the wound with Mercurochrome. He thought nothing about it. But six days later, his body ached frightfully, he couldn't move his legs and his jaws were stiff.

Douma figured he was done for. He had been a veterinarian and had seen animals die of lockjaw. Now he had it!

The farmer was "stiff as a chair" when his son lifted him into his car and took him to a clinic in Lansing. The doctors there agreed with Douma. He was dying of tetanus. They rushed him to the nearest hospital, about ten miles away—St. James.

Douma immediately was given standard therapy for tetanus—a tracheotomy (insertion of tube in his throat to facilitate breathing), tetanus antitoxin, sedation, muscle relaxants, and antibiotics. There was little chance he would survive. It was the moment to try to push the S.A. Healy people.

Pascale promptly phoned and talked to a Mr. Fields, the yard manager, who already was familiar with his requests for a tank. The doctor explained the urgent crisis.

"We want to do something now—and either yes or no," Pascale said. "I don't mean to put you on the spot because you people are evaluating it, and if it's no, that's all right with me, but if it's yes, I want to move. Because I may not have many more days with this patient."

"I understand," said Fields. "Give me till three o'clock. I'll give you an answer then."

At 2:30, Fields called to say he would send the 8 by 16-foot tank out next morning with a Healy crane to set it in place.

Next morning, May 31st, the tank was set in place on the parking lot close to the back wall of the hospital. Pascale and Wallyn were afraid it had come too late. Douma, no longer able to see or hear, was sinking fast.

There were other dark clouds; the tank was thirty years old and didn't seem fit to use. It was suitably divided into two compartments, but without lights, heat, or cooling, had no telephone for communication, and they oil seal leaked in the compressor.

"Listen, we can use flashlights," Pascale told Wallyn. "Hook up the compressor in our hospital laundry. Push those pipefitters to get on over here and make the connections. I'm going to call Boerema."

Pascal had never used hyperoxygenation, and he intended to ask the famous Dutch surgeon's advice.

From his office in Amsterdam, Boerma tried to be helpful. But, unfortunately, he had not yet treated tetanus in his hyperbaric chamber. He was, though, able to offer a few pointers and much encouragement.

Pascale hung up and went out to check progress on the tank. Kibitzers clustered around the boiler-like device. The pipefitters were on the job, but they estimated it would take eighteen to twenty-four hours to connect all the piping. The men agreed to work straight through until they finished.

Pascale went back to the phone and called Brown at Duke. Brown also was unable to offer any guidance, but added, "I think you're certainly justified in trying it." Wallyn and Pascale then found a Navy manual on submarine medicine and studied it.

The pipe fitters had the tank ready in 18 hours. The St. James doctors ran a couple of pressure tests, quickly got familiar with the controls, and then wheeled out the unconscious lockjaw victim and took him into the tank.

They clanged shut the doors, pressurized the old tank, and fed pure oxygen into Douma's lungs through his endotracheal tube. For a couple of hours, they anxiously watched him. Somehow, he seemed better. Then he was taken out and back to his bed, where he spent a comparatively quiet night. The following evening, he was again placed in the tank for a second treatment.

Next morning, Pascal felt Douma's neck. "Just feel this, Dick! The neck's supple. Douma's going to get well!"

Within two weeks, the farmer was back home. Pascale and Wallyn not only had won the race; their battered old jerry-rigged tank had saved a life!

Chicago's reporters picked up the story and gave it a splash, as did Time. There was such a to-do that the Saint James doctors a few weeks later in the Journal of the American Medical Association accused the press of "sensationalizing" the experimental treatment. "The newspapers," wrote Wallyn, "took this in their teeth and went wild. They've sensationalized, misquoted and fabricated."

Wallyn said the doctors had insisted their names not be used. "As far as I'm concerned, tetanus treatment is just a spectacular side effect of hyperbaric tank use," Wallyn said, in the Journal. "I'm looking forward to putting coronary patients in the tank, as well as using it to treat shock."

All this time, Bernhard had not been idle back in Boston. He had checked over the Harvard tank, secured a crew of experienced technicians and recruited interested assistant surgeons. They began a series of five hundred operations on animals. Doing these under hyperbaric conditions told Bernhard just how much extra time he could expect to get from hyperbaric oxygenation in the tedious repair of tiny malformed hearts. The risk was always high; most blue babies are critical at birth, facing death within hours or days, almost always within a year, because of transposed blood vessels or holes between heart chambers.

On December 7th, 1962, Bernhard was ready. His first feeble patient was wheeled into the chamber. Bernhardt's knife was sheer and steady. The pressurized oxygen sustained the flickering spark of life, giving him extra minutes so he could be more meticulous. Still, he had to work fast; and at last, he finished. The operation was a glorious success.

Bernhard brought more blue babies into the tank and all operations were successful. He reported his work before important surgical conventions and became the new "star" of hyperbaric medicine early in 1963.

This had been a fitting triumph for the squat little old Harvard tank—which now stood recognized as the tool that permitted the first hyperbaric blue-baby surgery in America. Yet, just short months after this day of glory, the Harvard tank played the most ignominious role of its long history.

Into that venerable tank, in August 1963, doctors took the dying newborn son of President John F. Kennedy—and asked for the impossible miracle.

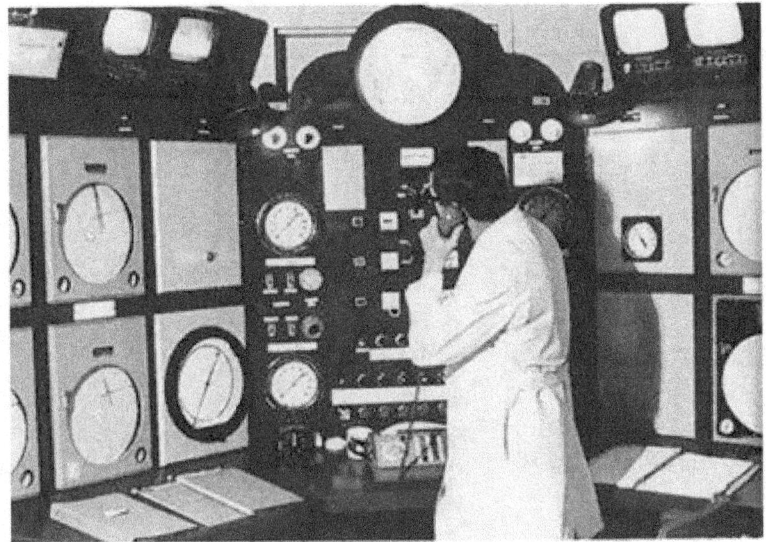

Control panel for twin chambers at St. Luke's Hospital, Milwaukee (Photo courtesy St. Luke's Hospital).

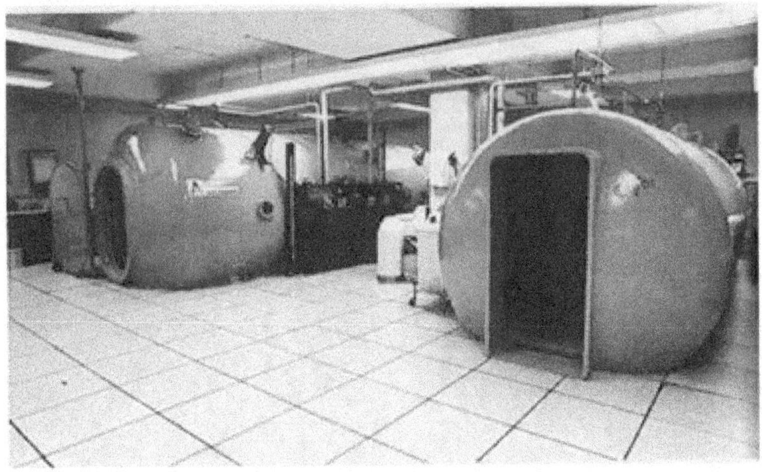

View of twin chambers "Bonnie" and "Clyde" at St. Luke's Hospital, Milwaukee (Photo courtesy St. Luke's Hospital)

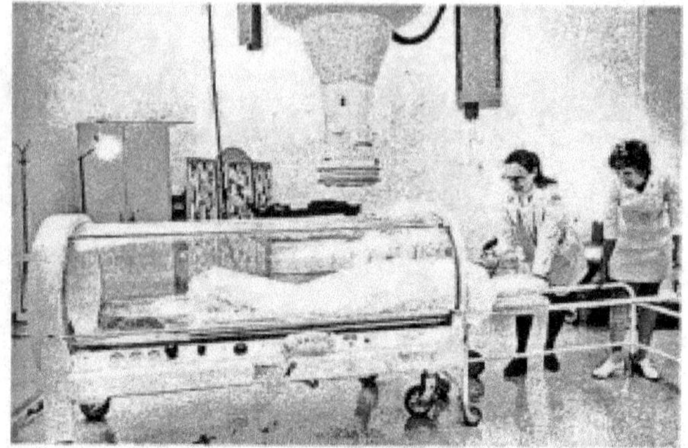

Dr. Cornelia Dettmer slides patient into Vickers chamber at Cincinnati's Christ Hospital. (Photo by Ranole Cochran)

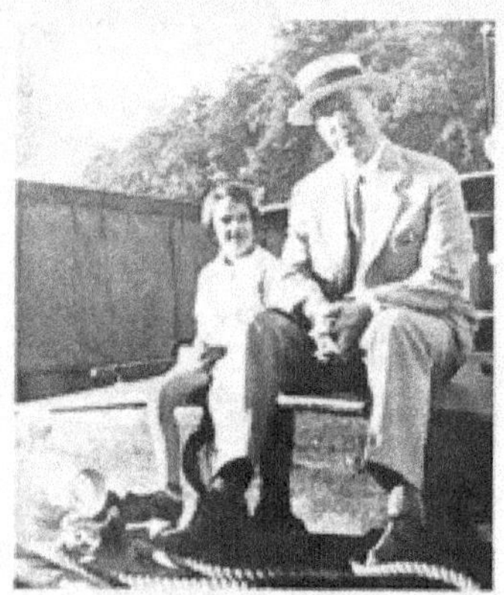

Dr. Cunningham and daughter Dorothy on hatch of his lake cruiser at Cleveland, circa 1929. (Photo courtesy the Cunningham family)

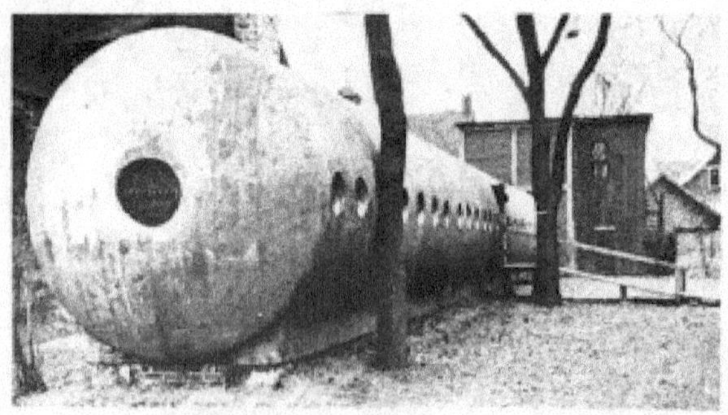

Dr. Cunningham's first tank on Harrison Avenue in Kansas City. (Photo courtesy the Cunningham family)

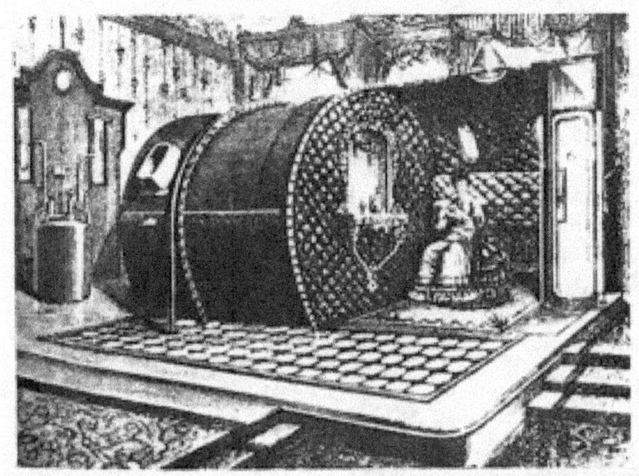

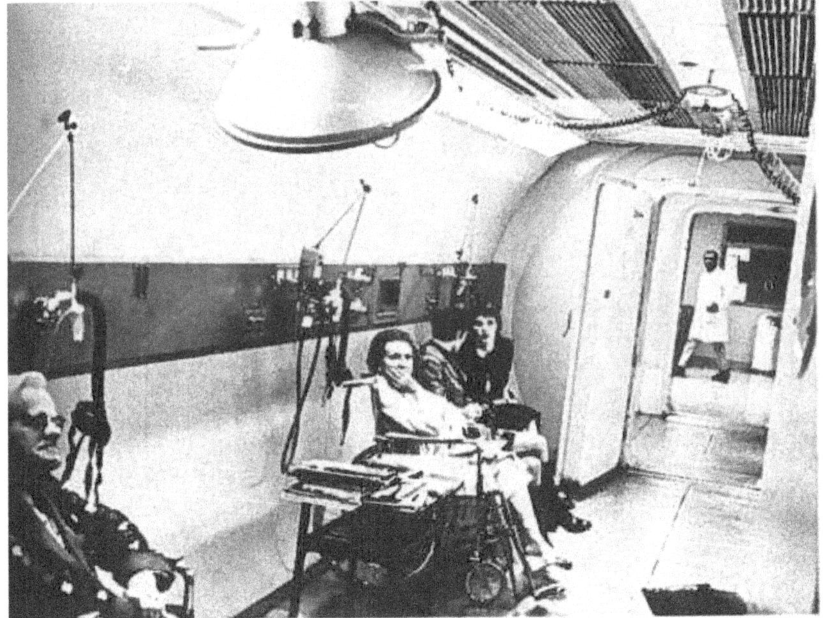

Inside one of twin chambers at St. Barnabas Medical Center, Livingston, N.J. Mrs. Thelma Segal, hand on chin. (Photo by author)

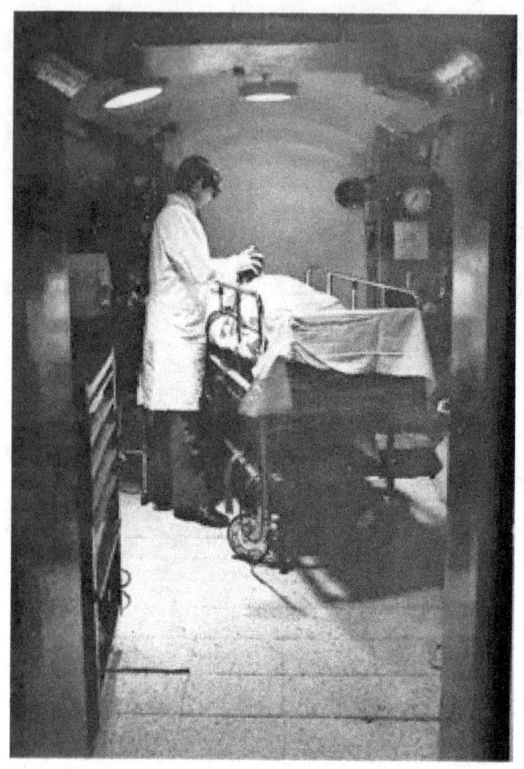

*Interior of chamber at St. Luke's Hospital, Milwaukee
(Photo courtesy of St. Luke's Hospital).*

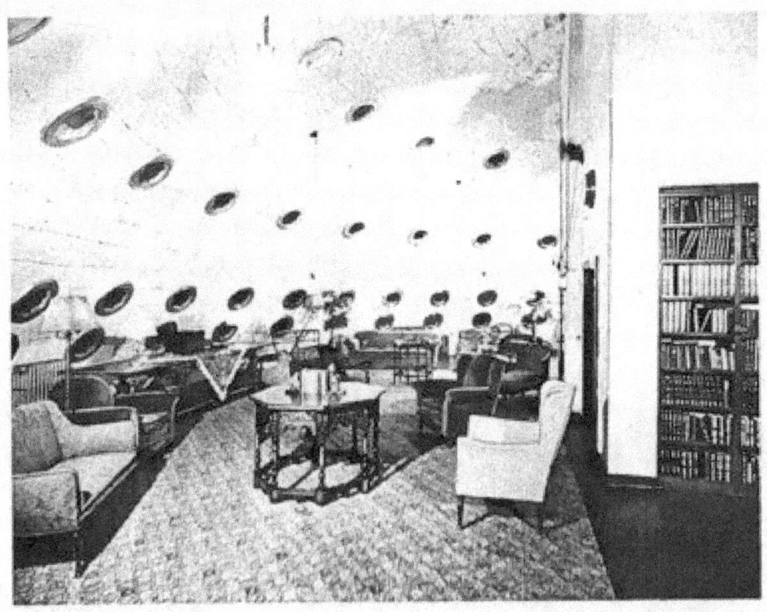

Lounge and reading room on top floor of steel-ball hospital in Cleveland. (Photo courtesy The Cleveland Press)

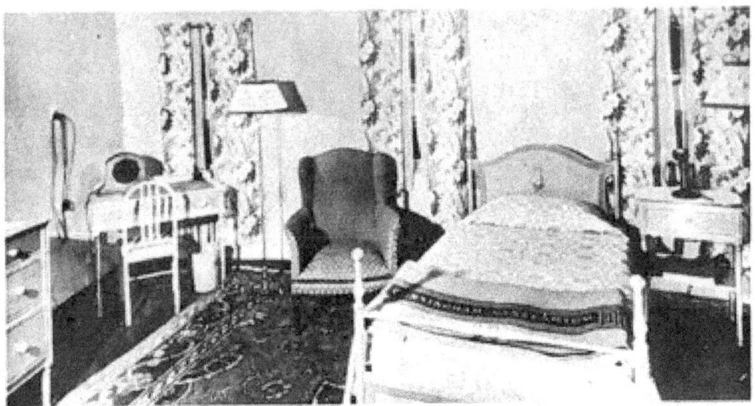

Bedroom inside the steel-ball hospital; note curtains covering portholes. (Photo courtesy the Cunningham family)

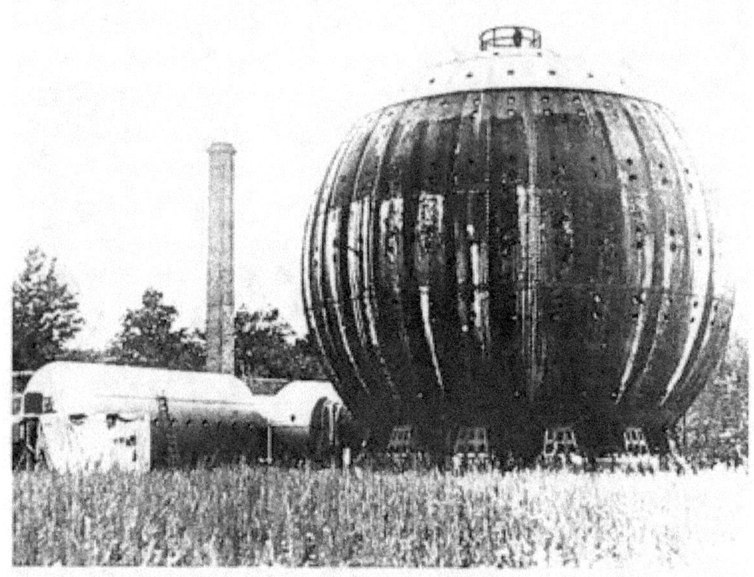

Steel-ball hospital and auxiliary tanks under construction. (Photo courtesy The Cleveland Press)

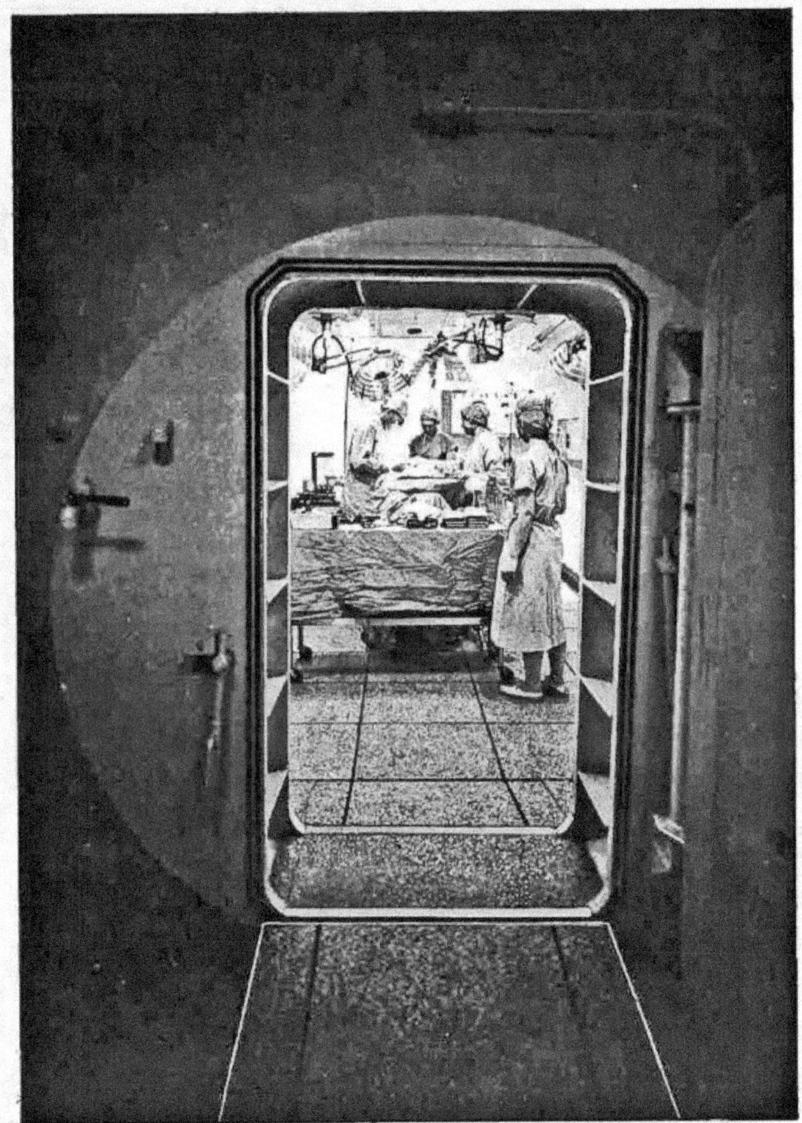

View through middle lock into operating room inside hyperbaric chamber at Lutheran General Hospital, Park Ridge, Illinois. (Photo courtesy Lutheran General Hospital)

6

PATRICK KENNEDY'S DESPERATE HOURS

Under the steamy blanket of late summer darkness, Boston squirmed and tried to sleep. It was after midnight and traffic should have thinned to a trickle in the Harvard Med hospital complex, but in these muggy first hours of Friday, August 9th, 1963, that section of Longwood Avenue was very much astir. A dozen police cars quietly prowled the avenue. Near intersections around Boston's world-famous 500 bed Medical Center lurked unmarked Secret Service sedans.

Lights blazed in the hospital's fifth floor nursery area and also gleamed in every basement window of the gray stone medical building that backs up to the hospital and faces 55 Shattuck Street. In the basement, in a small unpretentious room opposite the experimental dust chamber, stretched out shoeless and coatless on a hard-used leather couch, President John F. Kennedy slept uneasily.

At 2:10 am he was awakened. A doctor brought sad tidings—there was a definite change, for the worse.

The president went across the hall through a nondescript medical laboratory into the open door of a concrete block annex. Before him loomed a boiler-like white-enamel tank eight feet in diameter and thirty-one feet long, enmeshed in a strangling array of pipes, valves, and electric wiring. Electric motors hummed and the floor vibrated from the thudding of its air compressors.

The white-frocked technician scanning the large pressure dial squeezed forward to let President Kennedy slip behind him to get to a glass porthole.

Within the brightly lighted hyperbaric chamber, JFK saw five men in green surgical gowns and masks hovering over a gasping tiny infant—his newborn son, Patrick Bouvier Kennedy, at that moment barely thirty-seven hours old, and clinging to life by the most fragile thread.

The president leaned with one hand on the tank's enameled hull; he wondered at this contraption's sturdy bulk and simplistic mechanisms, while his reverie brought back the surge of optimism he had during the afternoon when the doctors first suggested that hyperbaric oxygenation might buy enough time for little Patrick to last out his crisis.

It would be a gamble they had said, but it was all they knew to do.

Jacqueline Kennedy had been vacationing since early July on Cape Cod with their two children, Caroline, five, and two-year-old John, Jr. Mrs. Kennedy was pregnant, but her baby was not due for six weeks and she planned to return in a fortnight to Washington in ample time to have her delivery at Walter Reed Army Hospital.

On Wednesday morning, August 7th, she left her leased house on Squaw Island in a car driven by a Secret Service agent and took her children to a riding stable seven miles away at Osterville.

Jackie, modish in a cream-colored shift and a jaunty straw hat, climbed out of the car shortly before 11 am and suddenly winced. There was a knife-like thrust in her side; she recognized the onset of labor pains. There was no time now for John-John and Carolyn to go horseback riding.

Immediately the car returned her to Squaw Island where also "vacationing" and standing by for just such an emergency were her obstetrician, Dr. John A. Walsh, of Washington DC, and the White House physician, Dr Janet Travell.

Walsh's quick examination confirmed that indeed the Kennedy baby was trying to arrive ahead of schedule. This did not surprise him nor his famous patient. Jackie had a long medical history of difficulties with pregnancies, beginning with a miscarriage in 1953.

Three years later—on August 23rd, 1956—she suffered an internal hemorrhage and lost her baby in the emergency Cesarean performed at the Newport, RI, hospital not far from her family's Hammersmith Farm home.

Then, hospital officials said the premature birth was brought on by nervous tension and exhaustion following the 1956 Democratic National Convention in which her husband had barely missed being made the Vice Presidential nominee. Later Mrs. Kennedy safely gave birth by Cesarean to her first child, Caroline, at a New York hospital November 27th, 1957. Then came the dramatic four weeks-premature birth of John, Jr., on November 25th, 1960, also by Cesarean section, at Washington's Georgetown University hospital after Kennedy's election as a president but before his inauguration.

Fortunately, on Cape Cod, everything to cope with another premature birth had been anticipated—and was in readiness. A special OB Suite was being held on standby for the First Lady at Otis Air Force Base in nearby Falmouth.

There was no delay. Jackie kissed her son and daughter goodbye. Walsh and a Secret Service agent escorted her and her secretary, Mary Gallagher, of Alexandria, Virginia, out on the lawn to board an Air Force helicopter, which immediately took off at 11:28 am for the 20-minute flight to Otis.

Travell went to the Secret Service trailer parked back of the Squaw Island house and picked up the ever-present direct line to the White House. Her call was put through to the president at 11:50 am while he was meeting with the Citizens Committee for a Nuclear Test Ban headed by James W. Wadsworth, former United States delegate to the United Nations.

Ambassador Wadsworth's group withdrew immediately. JFK summoned his personal secretary, Evelyn Lincoln, and Press Secretary Pierre Salinger to arrange a quick departure. Mrs. Lincoln began canceling the president's appointments. Salinger, perpetual cigar in hand, rushed to the lobby of the Executive wing to summon the wire service men and other White House reporters.

Bulletins were flashed out over the UPI and AP wires —the impending birth of a President's child is big national news. Reporters scrambled to get ready to accompany JFK to Cape Cod.

From the time Travell called, it only took seventeen minutes for President Kennedy to depart the White House. At 12:07 pm he was aboard his huge Air Force helicopter swooping off the South lawn with two Secret Service bodyguards, Mrs. Lincoln, and Salinger. At 12:30 their Lockheed Jetstar streaked off the Andrews runway. It would take the presidential party a good hour to cover the 450 air miles to Otis Air Force Base, on the southernmost tip of Cape Cod across the water from Martha's Vineyard.

Meantime Jackie's helicopter had landed at Otis at 11:48 am. A waiting ambulance whisked her to a suite in the nurse's cantonment. Then she was taken four hundred feet along an enclosed ramp to surgery.

Walsh, a pleasant, highly regarded then fifty-year-old capital "society doctor," began scrubbing for the operation. Four Air Force physicians joined him, along with a nurse captain and five medics. Walsh felt distinct apprehension. Preemies usually presented problems, this one—being almost five and a half weeks early—was virtually certain to emerge into the world with some kind of complication.

Walsh was not unduly worried about the mother. Jackie was then only 34 years old, with great stamina and in robust Health.

The Cesarean surgery began at once and went smoothly and quickly. At 12:52 PM Walsh delivered the First Lady of a son—well-formed, dark-haired, but only seventeen inches from toe to head and weighed a scant four pounds, ten and one half ounces.

Walsh carefully placed the infant in a waiting Isolette. The nurse slapped shut the transparent cover of the incubator, a three-foot square plastic box designed to bridge the gap between the mother's womb and the outside world, keeping temperature and humidity at the best balance to facilitate breathing.

For the moment that was all that could be done. The doctor maintaining the chart of the operation jotted down idiopathic respiratory distress syndrome—a smoke-screen term meaning difficulty in breathing for reasons unknown. The new Kennedy continued—even in this incubator's oxygen-enriched environment—to struggle for each puny breath. Wash saw serious trouble ahead.

At 1:28 pm, the Jetstar touched down at Otis and the president was taken straightway to the base hospital. A happy cheer came from the press and spectators. He turned, tanned and bear-headed, to acknowledge the good wishes with a wave of his arm. His sister, Jean Smith, who had heard the first news bulletin on her car radio while driving in downtown Hyannis Port, arrived at Otis in time to enter the hospital with the president.

Walsh came at once from surgery to inform the president of the conditions of mother and premature child, already routinely baptized by the base Catholic chaplain, Father John Scahill of Portland, Maine.

The president nodded his understanding; he and Jackie had decided in advance that if they had a son, he would be named Patrick (after JFK's immigrant grandfather) Bouvier (for Mrs. Kennedy's father, the late John V. Bouvier, who was a New York stockbroker).

Walsh explained that Mrs. Kennedy was fine, but the new son had some respiratory difficulty and was in an incubator.

At 2:10 PM Jackie returned to her suite. The president spent ten minutes with her—not mentioning anything about Patrick's trouble—and then returned to the surgical ward to get his first glimpse through the plastic incubator of his third child.

"A beautifully formed child," murmured the nurse. JFK grinned appreciatively.

Back in Washington, the Senate got the news when Majority Leader Mike Mansfield of Montana hurried down the aisle waving a bulletin torn off the UPI ticker and interrupted a debate to announce Patrick Kennedy's arrival. By coincidence, the baby's uncle, Senator Edward Kennedy of Massachusetts, was presiding. Senators broke into a loud cheer.

Within the hour congratulatory messages from chancelleries and world personalities began flooding the White House and Otis AFB. Everybody wished the newest Kennedy good fortune, good health, and a long life.

But the doctors at Otis observed that Patrick Bouvier Kennedy was weak and doing very poorly. At three o'clock Walsh drew the president aside and suggested calling a respiratory specialist from Children's Medical Center in Boston because of the possibility of hyaline membrane disease.

JFK seemed taken aback, apparently not having understood the serious implications. He told Walsh to do what the doctors deemed best.

In response to Walsh's phone call, the hospital authorities recommended Dr. James E. Drorbaugh, a quiet, 41-year-old associate in clinical medicine at Harvard. Within twenty minutes an Air Force helicopter swooped down into grubby little Fens Station in midtown Boston, not far from the medical center, to speed Drorbaugh to Otis. He found the infant in dire straits.

Little Patrick's shallow gasps for breath barely kept his lungs inflated and were overtaxing his tiny heart. The situation appeared critical. Drorbaugh recommended moving the infant to Children's Medical Center. There, he pointed out, a whole corps of specialists and all the latest modern medical facilities were available.

A flurry of telephone and radio messages set up police escorts along the sixty-seven miles the Air Force ambulance would travel to Boston.

But before departure, the President insisted, the First Lady deserved to see her newest child; and at 5:25 PM the Isolette was wheeled along the corridor to Jackie's bed. Through the plastic sides she had her first look at Patrick B. The president remarked casually about the breathing difficulty and offered optimistic comments on the impending transfer to Children's Medical Center.

At 5:50 PM began the dash by ambulance to Boston, behind siren-screaming motor cops. The outside world as yet had no inkling of the baby's serious plight. Someone at Otis asked a Secret Service man why the infant was being moved from the base hospital. "Oh," quipped the agent, "he's a Kennedy and dash they like to travel!"

While Walsh remained to attend Jackie, JFK boarded a helicopter at 6:18 pm and flew to the Squaw Island vacation house to tell Caroline and John-John they had a new brother, and to have dinner and rest briefly.

Exactly one hour later in Boston, nurses hanging out upper windows and a cheerful throng on Longwood Avenue heard the scream of sirens and broke into applause as the OTIS Air Force Base ambulance whirled up to the emergency entrance of the medical center's Farley Building. The rear door swung open, Drorbaugh leaped out with the medical charts and rushed inside. Captain William Jablonski carefully lifted out the Isolette. Some spectators and a few news photographers got a clear but fleeting view of the newest Kennedy, swathed in a blue blanket, his hair thick and long, lying on his stomach in the incubator. Captain Jablonski carried the precious package inside and took the elevator directly to a fifth floor suite opposite the nursery.

From that moment forward every resource of the vast medical complex was thrown actively into the battle for Patrick's survival.

Ten minutes after 8 that night the President returned to Otis by helicopter for a half-hour visit with his wife and then departed for Boston in his Air Force One Reserve backup 707 that had been brought up from Washington.

A little after nine o'clock, in surgical mask and gown, he was in room 2534, where specialists gathered around the Isolette evaluating the infant's prognosis. Present were half a dozen of the top men. X-rays had been taken and intravenous feeding started, the president was told; otherwise, there was no change in condition. Feeling reassured, the President left the hospital at 9:38 pm and went the Ritz-Carlton Hotel, where the Kennedy family maintained a year-round suite, and retired for the night.

What the medical experts were reluctant then to make clear to the President was their worry that Patrick was on the verge of hyaline membrane disease, the number one killer of newborn infants in the country, claiming an estimated 25,000 lives a year—mostly of premature babies.

The mysterious disease attacks the lungs of infants causing a glassy film to coat the lining of the tiny air sacs. This makes it difficult for the lungs to freshen the blood—to take out the gaseous carbon dioxide which should be exhaled and get full benefit from the nourishing oxygen being inhaled. The glassy film—hyaline comes from the Greek word for glass—stiffens the lungs. HMD is usually fatal in one of every two cases.

Pierre Salinger set up press headquarters in the Statler Hotel, where by now one hundred reporters had gathered, and by 10 pm was issuing a communique playing down the infant's plight. When asked if the baby was on the danger list, Salinger grunted, "I would not say that." He added that Patrick's malady was "not uncommon in premature babies." The rotund press spokesman, too, was hoping for the best.

Frankly worried, Drorbaugh refused to leave his famous little patient and sat with him through the night. About all the physicians could do was try to maintain the balance in Patrick's blood chemistry—and wait. If he could be kept going for 72 hours, the glassy film probably would evaporate. But it was clear the infant definitely was not getting enough oxygen into his bloodstream through his clogged lungs; and his gasping, fast breathing was dangerously straining his tiny heart.

Of a sudden, Drorbaugh thought of a brilliant colleague, Doctor William F. Bernhard, the 39-year -old Harvard surgeon who had just recently gained world attention by performing risky, delicate blue-baby heart surgery in Harvard's thirty-five-year-old hyperbaric tank. The pediatrician actually knew very little about the mystique of the pressure chamber; but first thing in the morning he'd ask Bill Bernhard if that tank would force more oxygen into the Kennedy baby.

Next day, Thursday August 8th, was overcast and sticky. At 9:45 am the President finished breakfast and drove to the hospital for a conference with Patrick's doctors.

At the same time the reporters at the hospital got Salinger to hold a press conference in which he conceded that the baby's condition was "still serious." That was the first ominous note to the public —the word "serious" had previously not been used. Fresh bulletins flashed this news across the country.

Something was broached to JFK in this morning medical huddle about the possibility of resorting to hyperbaric therapy. The president had been a Navy PT Boat Skipper in World War II and probably had seen diver-decompression tanks, but he had no substantial knowledge about the medical use of oxygen under pressure.

President Kennedy, anxious to keep his wife reassured and knowing that news accounts were now terming the baby's condition "serious," flew back to Otis at 10:30 am and visited Jackie before taking a helicopter to Squaw Island for lunch with his mother-in-law, Mrs. Hugh D. Auchincloss. His plans were to visit Jackie again at 4:00 in the afternoon and stop by the hospital in Boston at 6 o'clock.

During lunch, he got a phone call from Boston. The doctors were quite worried; little Patrick appeared to be slipping. The President said he would return at once. And at 2:15 PM, while firemen sprayed the Fens Stadium infield with fire hoses, his helicopter landed in a storm of dust which blinded the inevitable spectators. Mrs. Auchincloss and the President stepped out and went straightway to Children's Hospital.

A lengthy conference was held in Patrick's room. Finally, two decisions were reached. Mrs. Auchincloss engineered one. That was to try to bring in for consultation Dr. Samuel Levine, a famous New York specialist who had successfully presided over the survival of prematurely born Anna Christina Radziwill, the daughter of Jackie's sister, Princess Lee Radziwill.

The other decision was to ask Bernhard to try to work some magic by putting Patrick in the hyperbaric tank. That couldn't be done immediately; it would require time to round up technicians and get the seldom-used tank, located in the basement of the building directly behind Farley Building, ready for use.

There was one thing to understand, the president was warned. This would be strictly a gamble. There had been no specific use of a hyperbaric chamber to eradicate the glassy lung condition that anyone knew about. On the other hand, it did seem reasonable that the squeeze of the tanks compressed air might force enough oxygen into the tiny body to lessen the frantic struggle for each and every breath, and thereby relieve some of the burden on Patrick's straining heart.

Someone was busy on the phone trying to track down Levine in New York. The President and Mrs. Auchincloss went back to the Ritz-Carlton. And now, in mid-afternoon, began the desperate hours—and the gamble on the hyperbaric tank. Technicians began reporting to the basement of the Shattuck Street Building and checking out valves, wiring, compression, motors, and seals on the heavy iron doors.

It appeared Levine couldn't be found. He had retired as senior professor of pediatrics at NYU Cornell Medical Center and was somewhere wandering around Manhattan. Then at 3:55 pm he was located and instructed to go to Butler Aviation Terminal. There an Air Force Jetstar would be standing by to rush him to Boston.

Just about the time that he got there, Drorbraugh and Bernhard were having Patrick's Isolette brought from The Farley building down to the basement where the hyperbaric chamber now was in readiness.

Bernhard had assembled a corps of specialists, many of whom had some previous experience in the tank with animal experiments or his blue-baby operations. Jim Carr, who had been the technician for his previous work, was now handing out static-proof surgical gowns to the doctors and reminding them to take off their wrist watches (the crystals might pop out) and suggesting they practice popping their ears. Carr reminded Bernhard that a myringotomy should be done to equalize pressure on the baby's eardrums.

Bernhard explained to the other doctors it would be a matter of feeling their way and he could not estimate how long Patrick should be kept under pressure. Several were dubious about this desperate undertaking. However, they felt the hospital should be trying something—and up to now nothing at all seemed to enhance the outlook for survival.

At 4:41 pm the Isolette was carried through the iron doorway into the entry lock, and on into the No. 2 Compartment where the historic blue-baby surgery had taken place. The heavy doors were closed and dogged. Then the compressed air buildup begin with its gentle hiss.

On the intercom, Bernhard began monitoring readings with the console operator beyond the cylinder's iron wall. Drorbaugh and the others eagerly watched the jiggled lines on the cardiograph whose sensors kept track of Patrick's heart and respiration.

In a few minutes Drorbaugh pointed excitedly to the cardiograph. "Look at that!" The jiggles were indicating decreases in both heartbeat and respiration rate. "We may have something here!"

Only air was pressurizing the interior of the chamber, but by means of a flexible hose attached to an incoming supply line, 100% oxygen was being fed directly into the Isolette. And, indeed, very quickly the baby looked better. He was pinker. The miracle of the tank therapy actually was forcing more oxygen through his stiffened lungs into his starved blood.

This decision to resort to last ditch measures would remain for several more hours unknown to anyone except the hospital staff and the Kennedy family. The public was not told immediately about the use of the HBO tank.

While drama was unfolding inside the pressure chamber, Levine arrived on the scene. The distinguished consultant hopped out of the Air Force jet at Logan Airport into a waiting helicopter and was whisked to a dusty landing at Fen's Stadium. At 5:05 PM a police car delivered him to the hospital.

He could not, of course, examine the patient he had come to see. The New York specialist was a little flustered to find that the baby was in the oxygen chamber. He pored over the baby's chart and studied the x-rays. For half an hour he conferred with the physicians familiar with the case. He sadly shook his head. He was unable to suggest a better treatment. The last hope rested on the venerable Harvard hyperbaric chamber.

Outside the hospital a line of spectators doggedly hung on for a glimpse of any of the Kennedys, sympathetic but persistent—and specifically unaware of the desperate dice being tossed in the Shattuck Street basement.

Shortly after 6 o'clock Press Secretary Salinger broke the news about the hyperbaric chamber. He identified it as the only one in the United States, an understandable mistake.

The Press Secretary told how Levine had been flown up from New York. Then he fielded a barrage of questions. He understood the tank had been used 28 times with children.

"Were all those successful?" asked a reporter.

Salinger shook his dark head. "They were not all successful. I believe most of them were."

At this point a shout of "Thank you, Mr. Secretary!" broke off the press conference and triggered a mad scramble for phones. Most of the reporters were totally unfamiliar with hyperbaric—and were content to identify the Harvard tank merely as a high pressure chamber.

Inside the tank, the doctors were apprehensive. True, the pressured oxygenation had somewhat relieved the baby's struggle for breath; but was this enough relief to carry Patrick another 24 to 48 hours, the crisis period?

Attorney General Robert Kennedy and family aide Dave Powers flew up from Washington and joined the President in the room outside the tank about 8:30 pm. There was no good news. The distraught father was told candidly it was touch-and-go.

It looked like a long night; hospital administrators commandeered the doctor's lounge on the fourth floor of the Farley building and moved in a bed and television set for the president. He and Bobby stood outside the tank until the first medical team emerged at 9:05 pm to be replaced by the rotating crew of five others.

Then the two Kennedys and Dave Powers went to the fourth floor lounge to await the next medical conference at 11 o'clock.

Reporters were clamoring for an update, and Pierre Salinger gave them a briefing at 9:27 pm. He disclosed then that the first medical team had come out of the tank after spending four hours and twenty-four minutes with the baby and had been replaced by another team. He explained that the doctor teams would now rotate every two hours.

"The decision has been made by the doctors," Salinger said, "to keep the baby in the pressure chamber through the night." The President, he said, was waiting to talk with the physicians again at 11:00 and if there was no change in Patrick's condition would return to the Ritz-Carlton for the night.

The New York Times Reporter asked, "Would you still describe the baby's condition as serious?"

"I would."

"Pierre, are the doctors encouraged by this treatment?"

Salinger looked thoughtful for a moment. "Let me say for background that what is being done here has never been done before really, because this baby is suffering from a lung ailment, while the other babies who have been put in the chamber have all been operated on for heart problems. So, there is really no precedent for what is going on. That is not attributable to me by name—say sources or hospital sources."

The 11 o'clock medical report was discouraging. The president was told that his son's heartbeat was now very erratic. Bobby Kennedy and Dave Powers departed for the Ritz-Carlton, but JFK decided to remain near his son, not in the fourth floor doctor's Lounge, but in the basement room across from the tank.

He was deeply distressed by the harsh uncertainty. Frequently he would stride across the hall and squeeze up next to the tank to look in through the glass porthole. That intervals he collapsed onto the leather couch and stared blankly at the ceiling. Occasionally he would converse with doctors or the Secret Service men.

Finally—after midnight—he slipped off his jacket and loosened his tie. He took off his shoes and stretched out on the couch to try to get a few hours' rest.

At 2:10 in the morning he felt a hand on his shoulder, shaking him gently awake. He sat up and heard the doctor's heartrending message. No longer was there any hope at all. It was just a matter of time. Patrick was dying. His violent gasps for air were literally wearing out his tiny heart.

The President was pressing up against the tank peering in at the harried doctors, when Bobby Kennedy and Dave Powers got there. The President's brother said something meant to be consoling—but the impending loss was almost too much for either to bear.

Turning his head away, JFK went back and stretched out again on the couch. He couldn't sleep; he didn't feel like talking, not even to Bobby. He bowed his head and muttered a private prayer for his doomed son.

About twenty minutes before four, the president again squeezed up beside the porthole. Bobby looked over his shoulder. Inside the doctors continued to work feverishly.

At 4:04 am everything stopped. There was a stark sudden quiet. Drorbaugh recoiled from the Isolette, threw his hands over his gaunt face, and his lanky frame sagged in near total exhaustion.

Patrick Bouvier Kennedy was dead.

He had precariously lived for thirty-nine hours and six minutes in a world that seemed to promise him everything.

Medicine couldn't save him. Not even the sometime miracle of the hyperbaric chamber—which has given so much to so many lesser citizens—could guarantee this famous son of an American President his golden heritage.

7

AND THE BOOM GOES ON

A tragedy of the magnitude of the Kennedy baby's death might have been expected to put a fast damper on hyperbaric medicine. It didn't.

The wave of enthusiasm that had been building for so many months simply kept growing. The dreams and schemes of scores of alert hyperbarists were taking concrete shape—in the form of lavish money grants, the building of sophisticated and costly hardware, and more success and experimental work.

Hitchcock and Minneapolis had received the first federal grant ever awarded for construction of a hyperbaric chamber. Work began in June 1963 on his half-million dollar complex, with the National Institutes of Health contributing $237,839. This was going to be a first- class facility; the annual operating cost alone was estimated at $100,000.

Likewise, Van Elk had talked the John A. Hartford Foundation out of $490,000 to begin the big complex at Lutheran General Hospital in Park Ridge, the Chicago suburb, and construction began in June 1963. Eventually the Hartford Foundation put a total of $1,175,000 into it.

Duke Medical Center got a $386,058 grant from the National Institutes of Health and began building a five-chamber complex, four cylindrical tanks attached to a ten-foot sphere that served as an operating room, all of it forming a V.

The pioneering little tank at Saint James Hospital was kept busy treating tetanus and carbon monoxide victims. The McCormick Foundation gave $25,000 to fix it up. The Chicago Heart Foundation handed over $14,000 for experimental surgery that would permit photographing the inside of a beating heart. This was achieved by substituting clear synthetic plasma for blood in a dog, thus creating a clear visual field.

And by August 1964 Wallyn and Pascale could report in the Journal of the American Medical Association that at Saint James Hospital in nine patients with clinical tetanus there was active regression of symptoms following hyperbaric therapy. "The progression of the disease was arrested and reversed," they reported. "Seizures were reduced. The mental clarity and cooperation of these patients resulted in better control of respiratory problems and nutritional requirements. The need for tetanus antitoxin and tracheotomy was avoided."

Interest now was spreading worldwide. The First International Conference on Hyperbaric Medicine had been held in Amsterdam as an appropriate tribute to Boerama, with many Americans attending. Hitchcock, there to describe the tank being built in Minneapolis, read the conference a letter written by a woman who read about his federal grant in a Minnesota newspaper. She wrote:

"My heartiest congratulations for procuring funds for building of a hyperpressure chamber at General Hospital... this news has special significance to me. My leg was saved by tank treatments last May in Amsterdam. I was admitted to the hospital at night and treatment began the next morning. Gangrene had set in by the time I arrived there. I had ergotamine poisoning due to excessive use of Cafergot for migraine.

Previously to that night I had turned my foot in Paris, and it was examined there as a sprain. Dr Brummelkamp and Doctor Boerema diagnosed the illness. I am eternally grateful to them. They had used the tank for circulatory disease to a great extent but had not had a case previous to mine due to this drug.

I am recovering well. They had given up hope of saving the leg after the first three days; on the fourth day the temperature of the foot changed. I wish you much success in use of the tank. I might add that we were vacationing in Europe and were to leave for home from Amsterdam. We knew nothing of Professor Boerema or the tank. We went to Wilhelmina hospital because we were told we would get quick emergency treatment. Thus, it was all chance, and our very good luck!"

Not everyone was enthusiastic. Snide comments were voiced that HBO was on the verge of being a hospital status symbol. Even so, a real boom was on. Two hospitals on the West Coast joined the parade and ordered chambers. Presbyterian in San Francisco opted for $200,000 sphere 10 feet in diameter. The Hospital of the Good Samaritan in Los Angeles was acquiring a 10 by 30-foot tank for $50,000. And in Milwaukee, Saint Luke's was so impressed with the looks of the tank being finished by Allis-Chalmers that it put in an order for a second one, 8 by 20 feet, to be built by Biggs-United.

Such a widespread flurry of talk, action, and planning could be expected to alert the powerful "watchdog" over the American Scientific Community, the National Academy of Sciences—National Research Council. The big wheels in the academy couldn't sit idly by and risk letting any group of enthusiasts distort the effects of this new therapy. At the same time, if there had been a breakthrough, the National Academy should certainly try to guide these new medical efforts into the most productive and beneficial channels for the public good.

Eight physicians and one manufacturer, all of whom were considered especially knowledgeable in the field, were drafted by the committee on Shock, Division of Medical Sciences, to form the Ad Hoc Committee of Hyperbaric Oxygenation.

Dr. Alan Thal, who had tried using the submarine in the Detroit River on a sickle-cell patient, was chairman. Other members: Albert R. Behnke, George F. Bond, and Ralph W. Brower, Navy physicians with submarine medicine experience; Brigadier General Sam F. Seeley, former Chief Surgeon at Walter Reed Army Hospital in

Washington DC; three medical college professors, Brown of Duke, Cowley of Maryland, and Dr. Edward H. Lanphier, of the State University of New York at Buffalo; and John C. Carter, of the Linde Division of Union Carbide Corp.

For several months they inquired into what was being done and speculated on what should be done. Their work was finished by April 1963—several months before the Patrick Kennedy tragedy. They really had done an outstanding job of preparing a comprehensive white paper that accurately and fairly assessed the situation as it existed at the time and established practical guidelines for the future.

Their "Hyperbaric Oxygenation: Potentials and Problems" ran 14,000 words, and sounded notes of caution throughout lest hospitals and physicians overlook some problems in HBO. At the same time, the report read:

There is apparent justification for current enthusiasm, but to gain a worthy place in the therapeutic armamentarium the test of time will require that this modality must meet at least three criteria:

It must be uniquely beneficial, having clear-cut advantages over less formidable forms of treatment; it must be fully practical in its use in at least a few important conditions; and, in consequence trauma it must be applicable to a reasonable number of patients.

How well the clinical investigators met these criteria, the Ad Hoc committee warned, would determine whether HBO became available in hospitals throughout the world, or "is returned to that status it has occupied largely since it was first suggested in the 1600s."

The white paper suggested creation of a "central agency"—obviously within the federal government—that would keep HBO investigators current on all new developments and would rapidly accumulate and evaluate clinical experience and would help guide research projects to avert needless duplication.

This recommendation, which ten years hindsight verified as one of the most pertinent in the white paper, was not followed. However, a couple of years later a worthy venture to disseminate information was undertaken, a "newsletter" dreamed up and single-handedly carried on by Dr Harry J. Alvis of Buffalo, New York.

A former Navy submarine and diving medical officer and one of the leading HBO experts, Alvis maintains surveillance over hyperbaric chambers at two Buffalo hospitals, the Veterans Administration and Millard Fillmore. The first issue of his highly interesting quarterly was distributed in January 1965. It was a non-profit venture, and about 300 subscribers were on his mailing list at three dollars per year. In January 1973 Alvis's publication was merged into the Undersea Medical Society's newsletter Pressure, edited by Milwaukee's Eric Kindwall (six dollars yearly to non-members).

The white paper warns strongly against improvised or helter-skelter experimentation. The words did not dissuade aggressive investigators such as Van Elk at Parkridge's Lutheran General. In October 1963—just two months after the Kennedy baby episode and at least four months before his magnificent three chamber complex would be ready for use—a 12-year-old boy with a badly broken arm was brought to his hospital. The lad's hand was swollen with gas gangrene. Here was a life-or-death situation. The hand was already dead. Van Elk looked at the boy and shook his head sadly.

"If we could just somehow get this little fellow into a hyperbaric chamber," Van Elk lamented, "we might save him."

The doctor broke off and went down to the hospital basement and examined his Borg-Warner unit, a cylinder just 30 inches in diameter and 54 inches long, designed for animal experiments but in which he already had oxygenated three blue babies. He squinted inside and calculated the size of the 12 -year-old gangrene patient.

The boy was brought down to the chamber and carefully eased inside. With his knees bent over a small pillow, the boy would fit inside, and the door could be closed. He was given ten dives. The gas gangrene was stopped just above the wrist. The boy lost his hand, but his life was spared by this ingenious use of a little tank, and the amputation was held to a minimum.

The headline feature at many medical conventions in 1964 was—guess what! The Second International Conference was held in Glasgow, Scotland; and a two-day conference was staged by the New York Academy of Sciences. At the annual AMA convention in San Francisco physicians "jammed the auditorium" for a "Symposium of Hyperbaric Oxygen Phenomena." Boerema came from Amsterdam to speak.

It was the year of startup for many of the big new tanks. Lutheran General and Park Ridge held its dedication February 4th, 1964—with Boerema special guest. And the Minneapolis General Hospital chambers went into use May 1st, after 18 months of work and expenditure of $526,000. Duke began using an 8 by 22-foot tank, the first unit of its complex. In Buffalo, New York, both Millard Fillmore and the Veterans Administration hospitals acquired 8 by 20 foot tanks. Chicago's Edgewater Hospital installed a similar chamber.

Hardly any doctor was more eager to get into clinical experimentation in a chamber than Cowley at the University of Maryland. But it seemed that every time he took one step forward, he somehow was propelled back two or three.

First his ill-fated attempt to take an 8 by 39-foot fiberglass cylinder and convert it into an HBO tank. The tube was made by Hercules Powder Co. as a sample container for a solid fuel booster being considered for the Saturn moon launcher. When NASA opted for liquid fuel to propel man to the moon, Hercules had no need for the sample.

Cowley thought the ends could be closed up and it would make a fine pressure chamber, and perhaps it would have. Hercules presented it as a gift, a trucking company hauled in the plastic tube and set it in place at the medical school. Cowley's men fitted doors on each end and concealed compressors. The doctors were all smiles, hardly able to wait their chance to get inside and try to establish a few new medical milestones.

First the tank had to be tested. Cowley's crew pressurized the tank to 2,000 PSI and left it overnight. Next morning the gauge read 75 PSI! What had happened? Cowley couldn't understand. They repeated the test. Next morning the gauge needle again was down to 75.

The dismayed Cowley undertook a very thorough check. Inside the tank he could see scratches, gouges, and a tiny break in the fiberglass lining. By deduction it was then clear that somewhere in the loading, moving or unloading process some careless rigger had inserted timbers into the open ends of the cylinder and attached his hoisting cables to them.

The loose timber ends jiggling inside had done the dirty work. The minute ruptures made the tank totally unusable; the leaks couldn't be safely repaired. There was no way to discover who was guilty of abusing the tank, and it was abandoned.

Then Cowley attended the Glasgow International Conference and was not favorably impressed with the Scots' crude chamber.

Undaunted, he sought out Jerome Touhy of Baltimore's Dixie Manufacturing Company, who had a lot of experience in building pressure tanks. Cowley gave him a spiel from his heart about contributing to mankind's need, and pointed out that if Dixie built Maryland University a good tank it might well serve as a showpiece for future sales. Touhy was a pushover—and, Cowley says, a hell of a nice guy. He built Cowley a chamber at actual costs; meaning about $20,000 for a tank that would retail for 50,000 to 70,000.

But the Maryland experimenter's elation at getting the Dixie tank was unfortunately quickly dashed. Maryland University was in the midst of a building program in Baltimore. Somehow the contractor got crosswise with the federal government, and everything came to a grinding hall for about two years.

The nation's boilermakers were eyeing the HBO developments more eagerly than a kid at a Christmas toy counter. Business Week reported in February 1964 that manufacturers saw production of these chambers as a possible $25,000,000 annual market. If the inherent promise of HBO "in treating coronary attacks and open heart surgery should work out," said the magazine, "the market for the chambers would include at least 200 general hospitals having 200 or more beds." The estimate was they might spend $100,000 each.

The industry was much too optimistic. Between the first of 1965 and the end of 1970 only seven hospitals installed major hyperbaric machinery.

Mount Sinai Hospital in New York City, where Dr. Julius H. Jacobson II has worked diligently at trying to prove the effectiveness of oxygenation, opened a 12 by 45-foot chamber February 2nd, 1965, with a smaller separate recompression chamber, 6.5 by 16 feet. Saint Luke's in Milwaukee dedicated its two tanks in 1966, and in the same year Saint Barnabas Medical Center at Livingston, New Jersey, put in use twin tanks 12 by 45-feet, and Children's Medical Center in Boston opened its complex consisting of a 16-foot sphere for surgery and a 9 by 28-foot medical tank.

New York University Medical Center opened in 1967 its three-chamber complex, all 10 feet in diameter and 8, 14.5, and 7.5 feet in length. The University of Pennsylvania got into the swim in 1968 with a $500,000 battery of four tanks, including a wet pot for physiological stress experiments for very deep saturation diving. And Maryland's Cowley finally started using his chambers in 1970, two tanks 10.5 by 52 feet and 6.5 by 17 feet.

Additionally, twenty to thirty single-patient chambers were installed in hospitals across the land for clinical research and treatment. Several strictly experimental research units also were built.

So finally, at long last, the parade has gone off and left behind the rugged little Harvard tank that made so much history on its own.

It is idle now. No one has used it for better than five years —for any purpose. In March 1972, William Keith, associate in physiology at Harvard School of Public Health, scrounged the keys, opened doors, snapped on lights, and let me step over some litter and inspect the interior of the historic chamber. I would not want to take a dive in it. Even in untrained eye can see it is unsafe, a fire trap.

That, in fact, is also the firm opinion held by the informal "chamber group" in the Department of Physiology. After a long study of the tank, Keith joined Dr. David E. Leith and three others in making a recommendation to Dr. James L. Wittenberger, department chairman. They suggested the tank was unsafe for their use.

Their communication dated March 26th, 1970, said in part:

"De-rating is recommended because we feel the facility and its operations are unsafe. The chamber presents grossly unacceptable fire hazards (for example, linoleum floor, Celotex subfloor, deteriorated insulation and "informal" wiring, exposed light bulbs, soldered oxygen piping{!}) paint of uncertain origin, and wooden fittings and other serious safety hazards (for example, poor communication with tenders, uncertain emergency power and air supply, lack of adequate provision for treatment of decompression accidents, and antiquated valving). The operation of the facility is casual; no individual exercises authority and has responsibility for its safety; no medical examination is required prior to entry; insufficient personnel are available for emergency staffing..."

It would cost $150,000 to bring the Harvard tank up to present safe standards. And with the gleaming new triple-chamber complex in Children's Medical Center standing idle much of the time now, it seems unlikely Harvard will decide to modernize the old tank.

It is a shame that the fabulous steel ball is gone. The Miriam Smith Rand tank should be saved—not for use, but as a relic of our medical history. Harvard should offer it to the Smithsonian Institute in Washington.

8

SURGERY, HEART ATTACK, CANCER, AND GANGRENE

Surgery

50 years ago, a surgeon needed little more for an operation than a kit of instruments and someone to drip ether on gauze over the patient's nose and mouth. Today's open heart surgery and organ transplants require operating room teams of a dozen specialists and batteries of instruments ranging from heart lung machines and artificial kidneys to recorders that monitor breathing, pulse and brain waves.

The hyperbaric chamber takes the surgeon even one further step. It makes possible, or at least safer, operations previously considered too risky. The tanks squeeze virtually guarantees that the patient's body will not be starved for oxygen. This has always been a big danger when the surgeon interrupts blood flow, especially to the brain.

The tank actually becomes the operating room and has been successfully used in surgical repair of congenital heart defects, aortic aneurysms, occluded carotid arteries, crush injury of the extremities, brain trauma, skin grafts, and detached retinas. HBO also has improved conditions for harvesting organs from cadavers and storing and transplanting them; and for making possible surgery on older patients who had been considered inoperable. It also markedly increases the effectiveness of heart-lung machines, and of hypothermia, body cooling.

Hyperbaric surgery was not undertaken in the United States until 1962, six years after Boerema's blue-baby operations in

141

Amsterdam. Bernhard of Boston Children's Medical Center was, of course, the American pioneer. Working in the cramped little Harvard tank on infants with malformed hearts, he undertook to confirm that HBO would provide a greater margin of safety in these high risk operations.

Seven thousand blue-babies were then dying annually in the United States, and surgeons had a terrible batting average on those they tried to salvage. For example, of 130 such patients operated on at Boston Children's between 1957 and 1962, only 60 survived surgery. It was often lack of oxygen that caused death—hypoxic cardiac arrest—before the surgeon could complete the tedious repair.

Bernhard first operated with HBO on dog hearts. Then he made safe experiments on sick infants by giving them oxygen during dives lasting one to three hours. The oxygen level went up as long as the baby was in the tank and dropped when it was decompressed. This convinced Bernhard that operating under pressure could guarantee enough extra oxygen to increase survival rates.

And he proved it. Of the first 135 blue babies he operated on in the Harvard tank, 110 lived!

The National Heart Institute was so impressed with the improved mortality rate that it gave Bernhard $339,500 with which to build at Boston Children's a magnificent hyperbaric complex. It consists of two large pressure chambers, one a circular operating room that easily accommodates a 12-man team. Bernhard's enterprise also won over the John A. Hartford Foundation, which gave him $467,520 to finance three years of clinical research.

Since 1962 hundreds of operations have been performed on humans in the hyperbaric tanks scattered across America. And thousands of others have been done experimentally on research animals, trying to confirm or expand clinical impressions in this relatively new field.

The first to employ a chamber as an operating room to repair aortic aneurysms was Jacobson, eminent vascular surgeon at New York's Mount Sinai Hospital. An aneurysm is the extremely dangerous ballooning of a weakened blood vessel. It may rupture in a fatal hemorrhage, especially if arteries near the heart or in the abdomen are involved. The weakened section is cut out and replaced with Dacron tubing.

As expected, the chamber pressure maintained a higher than normal oxygen level in the blood to the patient's legs during the minutes the big artery was clamped off. But Jacobson was surprised, and pleased, to discover it was possible to release the clamps immediately instead of having to do this in gradual stages over a period of about 10 minutes to avoid a serious low blood pressure complication called hypotension.

Jacobson, at the Third International Conference at Duke University, observed that "I am not saying this kind of surgery should not be done outside the chamber. But there is no question in my mind, on the basis of our first 50 cases, that it does add a measure of safety for the patient." Lanphier of Buffalo, New York, who was chairman of that particular discussion said, "The percentage of safety for the patient may not be very great, but if I happen to be the patient, I think I would prefer to chance Dr. Jacobson's method."

A hard blow to the head may dent the skull and pinch off the blood supply to the adjacent area of the brain. Interruption of circulation causes anoxia, a lack of oxygen. This produces swelling, which blocks even more blood vessels, and a vicious cycle is started that can lead to brain damage or death.

Jacobson treated a New York teenager hurt in an auto accident whose brain had puffed up so much that other surgeons had had to remove part of the boy's skull to allow for expansion. To avoid more swelling, he was put in the Mount Sinai chamber. That stopped the swelling at once. In fact, within 30 minutes the brain had shrunk two inches. The significance of this is clear in view of the vast number of head injuries caused by traffic accidents.

One common cause of stroke is a blood clot blocking one of the four carotid arteries which run up the neck to supply the brain. At Saint Barnabas Medical Center, a young New Jersey surgeon, Dr. Dennis R. Filippone, explained to me how the hyperbaric tank greatly lessens the danger of an operation to clear an included carotid artery, which requires such speed and skill it is known as "the surgeons nightmare."

Normally a surgeon would insert a small bypass tube into the artery on either side of the blockage to maintain blood flow and then clamp off the area in between he intends to operate on.

But use of such a tube has many shortcomings. Filippone points out it may get in the surgeon's way, or be too small to carry inadequate blood flow, or let air bubbles leak into the circulation.

Doing the surgery in a hyperbaric chamber means that Filippone could expose the artery and freely and safely put a clamp across it.

"This is unheard of," explains Filippone. "You're not supposed to do that. And we operate on this very leisurely, nothing in our way, and we do a good job."

While the operation proceeds, the surgeon inserts a small instrument into the adjacent vein to constantly monitor the amount of oxygen in blood that is returning from the brain. Surprisingly, says Filippone, this oxygen level is even higher than in arterial blood going to the brain of the average person. Thus, the patient with the clamped artery is perfectly safe due to the hyperoxygenation drenching effect.

"We can literally operate on such a patient for as long as we want and not worry about it," says Filippone. "No longer is the limit four minutes; we can take two hours if we need it."

Filippone cited two cases in which use of the chamber made possible operations on a woman of seventy-three and a man of eighty, both poor risks because of age. An aortic aneurysm obstructed the woman's throat; she couldn't eat. In an ordinary operating room, a catheter would be inserted into her heart to take blood out through a roller pump and return it through a vein in her leg. This bypass would permit the aorta to be clamped off so the diseased section could be replaced but this could reduce the oxygenated blood flow to the kidneys and spinal cord, endangering both; and would add the great risk of open heart surgery as well.

Filippone eliminated all this. He just put the woman in the chamber and clamped her. He monitored the oxygen to see that her kidneys were getting enough and was able to sew in a graft in a very brief period of clamping. She was out of the hospital in 10 days. Undergoing the same operation normally, a twenty-five-year old man might require a month to recover, the surgeon says.

The octogenarian had been bedridden for three months with prostatic obstruction necessitating continual catheter care drainage and was paralyzed on his left side. Surgeons didn't like the idea of operating because he also had congestive heart failure. However, they finally performed a cryo-surgical prostatectomy in the tank. Immediately after coming out of the anesthesia, the old man was able to move his paralyzed arms and hand. He walked out of the hospital and lived comfortably for seven months, at which time he died of congestive heart failure.

Hyperbarists are aware of one unusual hazard in their work—that long exposure to compressed air may intoxicate them. The effect is known variously as "raptures of the deep," "nitrogen narcosis," or "the martini effect." It is a kind of euphoria that develops gradually as a result of excess nitrogen.

In large tanks, only the patient is fed 100% oxygen, through either a face mask or an endotracheal tube; but the fact that the atmosphere is compressed to around 3 ATA means that the surgeons and technicians are effectively getting about 60% oxygen in the air they breathe instead of the normal 21 percent.

Within a few hours this can bring on a real jag. At the New York Academy of Sciences first HBO Symposium one physician spoke candidly about his personal experience with the problem. As reported by the Medical World News (March 13th, 1964):

An insight into the strange world of medicine at high pressure was provided by one speaker who described how, after being under six atmospheres for an hour, he was unable to distinguish between a hypodermic syringe reading of 1.25 cc and 125 cc.

At a Connecticut Hyperbaric Symposium, I asked an experienced anesthetist from New York if she had been bothered by the "martini effect." At once she said no. Then she thought it over and, with a wry smile, said: "Well, sometimes in the tank when I tear open the sterile box to take out a syringe, I find myself standing and looking down, trying to decide which I'm supposed to throw away—the box or the syringe."

Duke University's Brown believes that "Four atmospheres is about the upper limit for the surgical team breathing air to remain sufficiently sober to operate." Only rarely are doctors or nurses required to remain inside longer than an hour or two.

Occasions of long confinement usually involve the 38 hour procedure for reducing an air embolism, treating the bends, or a blood loss anemia case. In these instances, nobody takes any chance the "martini effect" will cause a tragic mistake. A supervising surgeon is posted on duty outside the tank, where he is not influenced by the high-pressure environment, and he monitors the activities inside by observation through portholes or TV cameras and consults via intercom. He either calls the shots or confirms decisions to guard against any erratic move by a member of the inside team.

Surgery in a hyperbaric chamber usually requires a larger staff, is not at all convenient, may take more time because of decompression, and subjects the whole team to the danger of the bends, especially if more than one operation a day is to be done. Because of cramped space, a small contoured operating table with a small base is used. Clothing, drapes, and linen must be pretreated to render them non-flammable, which produces a minor problem because of reduced absorbency.

Aqueous disinfectants are used for skin preparation to prevent the explosive vapors of alcohol from entering the chamber atmosphere. Saline is used to inflate endotracheal balloon cuffs, and intravenous fluids usually are administered from plastic bags instead of bottles.

There hasn't been a wild boom in hyperbaric surgery, but it is still used. And leaders in the field like Jacobson believe it has proved its merit and will continue to be employed in certain operations until an improved heart lung machine is developed that will more efficiently oxygenate a patient.

Heart Attack

Doctors remain greatly at odds over use of hyperbaria in heart attacks. Some clinical tests have been excellent (especially in London) but others have not increased survival rates. As in so many other areas of HBO, conclusive studies are needed to prove or disprove its effectiveness in this disease.

This is no minor controversy because heart attacks strike one million Americans a year, killing 675,000 — more than the combined annual total of the next three most prolific killers — cancer (325,000), stroke (210,000), and accidents (130,000). The commonest cause of death today is the so-called "coronary"— occlusion of a coronary artery which cuts off blood to the heart wall muscle causing a myocardial infarction, or destruction of a patch of the myocardium (heart muscle), which dies for want of oxygen.

Two major risks to life immediately haunt this patient: first, that the infarct will disrupt the nerve system that controls the heartbeat and will trigger a fatal arrhythmia (spasm that stops the pumping), and second, the effects of impaired circulation.

Dr. C. J. Gavey, head of the cardiac department at London's Westminster Hospital, explains that thus begins a vicious cycle. The rest of the myocardium is trying to compensate for the area that gets no blood, and hence no oxygen. But this attack usually causes the heart to slow down and pump less blood, which means the lungs can't do full duty. So even smaller than normal amounts of oxygen are reaching the unimpaired heart muscles. And that isn't all the bad news. The poor circulation triggers a metabolic crisis elsewhere in the body that even further hampers the damaged myocardium.

To Gavey and his associates this looked like a ready-made situation for applying HBO. That definitely would put more oxygen into the patient's blood. In theory it should send oxygen through the unblocked vessels to the ischemic (oxygen starved) tissues at the edge of the infarct area, preventing the impending death of additional heart muscle. That is doubly important; for within the hypoxic borders of the infarct area exists mechanisms believed to trigger fatal arrhythmias.

Of heart attack patients who reach the hospital, about 25 percent die within six weeks. The most critical period is the first twenty-four to forty-eight hours. Gavey decided to treat victims of heart attacks in his one-man Vickers chamber, pressurizing them at 2 ATA in 100 per cent oxygen for two hours, followed by a rest of one hour in plain air, and then continue the cycle of two hours in the pressurized chamber in one hour out for about four days.

Forty patients aged thirty-five to seventy-two, who had suffered a serious attack within twenty-four hours were treated in 1968-69. Thirty-seven survived the treatment, giving an immediate mortality of 7.5 per cent, but three of those died later (8 to 15 days) before leaving the hospital, giving a total mortality of 15 per cent.

Twenty-three of the patients arrived in severe pain and fourteen had difficulty breathing. Once inside the tank the patient no longer felt pain, and in thirty minutes any breathing problem was eased.

Publication of the Westminster Hospital results stirred a controversy. Scottish Physicians had four years earlier found no benefit at all in using HBO against myocardial infarction. They administered 100% oxygen by masks to twenty patients under pressure in a large tank. Twenty "controls" were given conventional treatment. The doctors in Scotland observe that the mortality rates had been identical.

Westminster Hospital, however, continue to run tests, and by the end of October 1970 had compared a total of 127 patients. Of 58 given hyperbaric treatment, 11 died, a mortality of 19%. Of 69 "controls," seventeen died, a mortality of 24.6%.

In comparison, the death rate overall in the hospitals entire coronary care unit was only 16% in 1970. The explanation offered for the higher mortality figures in the test program was that it included only the really critical cases.

Although need for still further tests was indicated, Westminster thought HBO was overall "beneficial." The treatment obviously saved some patients from fatal cardiogenic shock—all seven of their "controls" who were in shock died, as did but three of the six in the HBO group. It also was considered significant that in most of the serious cases, half of the "controls" but only 25% of the pressurized patients died.

At the 1970 Western Hyperbaric Medicine Conference at Good Samaritan Hospital in Los Angeles, a panel of experts tried to resolve the issue—and couldn't. As reported by Alvis in his Hyperbaric Medicine Newsletter (May 1970):

"The members of the panel displayed a degree of unanimity.... That was surprising in view of their diverse origins and areas of interest.

There seems to be general agreement on these points: that myocardial infarction is not a single disease, that there are good theoretical and experimental reasons for expecting hyperbaric oxygenation to benefit selected cases of infarction, that the problem is selection, and that in any clinical trial, treatment should be applied to controlled, rigidly defined and carefully selected clinical subgroups. The optimum hyperbaric regimen for this disorder has yet to be defined."

Cancer

In theory hyperbaric oxygenation should help radiation fight cancer. This is why: malignant tumors are laced with clusters of anoxic cells that strongly resist the destructive (and hence in this case curative) radiation which oxygenated cells accept. So if these oxygen-starved tumor cells were drenched, should they not respond more readily to X-rays?

The first "yes" came from Dr. Ian Churchill-Davidson of London's St. Thomas Hospital. He began in late 1954 treating a group of patients using radiation on one half of a large tumor in normal air, and then the other half of the cancer while the patient breathed 100% oxygen at 3 ATA. Later the tumors were examined by a pathologist who found more recognizable damage in the oxygen-treated half in seven of eight patients.

With this encouragement, Churchill-Davidson began extensively treating entire cancers. During the next ten years he found that oxygen-treated patients stayed free of a recurrence twice as long as those treated in air. There were some disappointing side effects. When X-rays were used on the larynx, sixteen of ninety-six developed radionecrosis of the laryngeal cartilage or destruction of part of the windpipe—and this happened only under HBO condition. However, this drawback later was overcome by reducing the X-ray dose.

Of more concern was that in 60 of 235 oxygen treated patients the cancer spread to another part of the body; but this ratio (26%) turned out to be about the same as in air-treated patients)30%).

Winnipeg General Hospital physicians found local tumors responded 45% better under oxygen and improved only 20% in air therapy but these doctors were dismayed to discover that in six of the HBO patients the cancer spread elsewhere and caused death within seven months. Only one of five in the control group died of cancer spread within 15 months.

At the University of Wisconsin Medical School, Dr. D. A. Tobin found his results were even-Stephen after a two-year comparison of air and oxygenated radiation. His experiments were terminated by the unfortunate explosion of his one-patient chamber (see details in Chapter 13) both doctor and patient were injured but survived.

Hundreds of other researchers have reported mixed success and failure. Extensive tests were still underway in 1973—including a major undertaking at Houston's MD Anderson Cancer Hospital. But leading radiologists expect no definitive conclusion in the United States until a national randomized series is run with all hyperbarists using identical modes of treatment.

Gas Gangrene

This is a savage disease, so rare that a doctor may encounter but one case in his career. Yet—until hyperbaric therapy was thrown against it in the 1950s—the attack usually killed its victim or left him maimed. It can erupt in ordinary wounds of violence—such as a fractured arm or leg or devitalizing crush injury sustained perhaps in a traffic accident. It may start when a woman bungles a self-abortion at home, or from bowel surgery in a sterile hospital operating room or even from a procedure as routine as an appendectomy.

Once the anaerobic gangrene bacillus Clostridium perfringens attacks, doctors are in a minute-to -minute fight against death. These vicious bugs are always around and waiting—lurking in the soil, on our skin and clothing, in food. They inhabit a healthy person's gastrointestinal tract. At death they are the putrification agents that form gas to help decay the body.

The gas-gangrene bacteria can invade tissue whose oxygen content drops to a low level. They multiply at a furious rate. A characteristic of such growth is the formation of a toxin which can kill and actually dissolve the cells—particularly muscle cells. Gas is formed as a byproduct of the rotting away of the dead cells. As these products of cell death and dissolution are absorbed, the patient becomes septic with local pain, high fever, and general debility.

As poison breaks down adjoining healthy flesh, the disease advances like wildfire, enlarging the wound, dumping more poison into the bloodstream and beginning to cripple the entire body.

The only practical treatment, before hyperbaric treatment, was surgery—speedy and drastic amputation! It was the only way surgeons knew how to jump ahead of the raging infection. If the gangrene was in the wrist, they reasoned, amputate at the elbow; in the forearm, amputate at the shoulder. Often even this was not enough. Penicillin came into use after World War II, yet massive doses cured only mild infections of gas gangrene. Once gangrene advanced beyond the shoulder joint or the hip, it was curtains for the unfortunate patient.

Use of hyperbaric oxygen—usually applied at 3 ATA—has prompt effects upon the organism, slowing its growth, and apparently stopping the formation of dreaded toxin which causes the cellular destruction. Comatose patients may wake up a few minutes after going into the tank. With treatment for five to ten days, eight out of ten victims recover. And instead of automatically losing a leg up to the hip the patient might get by with amputation of just part of a toe.

First use of hyperbaria against gas gangrene in the United States came in the fall of 1963. It dramatically saved the life of a 17 year old blonde co-ed at the University of Massachusetts.

The crisis arose out of a humdrum appendectomy. Sandra Olson felt the classic pain in her right side. When it began to really bother her the trouble was diagnosed, and an emergency operation was performed at Cooley Dickinson Hospital in Northampton to remove her ruptured appendix. Three days later, on September 22nd, her surgeon, Dr. David Jackson, checked the incision—was floored by what he saw. A telltale bronze patch spread across her abdomen, the wound gave off a foul odor, and the girl was feverish and in pain.

At once Jackson gave her gas-gangrene antitoxin, plus heavy doses of tetracycline and 12,000,000 units daily of penicillin. He took her to surgery and cleaned the wound, trimming away all the Flesh and muscle that was black and dying. But that didn't stop the deadly infection; within two days it had spread to her back. All the muscle on the right side of her abdomen was gone and half on her left side had been destroyed.

She was dying.

By a stroke of luck, the surgeon's wife, Patricia, had been a nurse at Boston's Children's Medical Center, where Bernhard one year earlier had done blue-baby surgery in the Harvard Medical school's hyperbaric chamber. She recalled that to her husband—and it was fresh in her mind that the tank had also been more recently used (August 1963) to try to save President Kennedy's infant son.

An ambulance rushed Sandra to Boston. Bernhard and the tank were waiting. Assisted by five other doctors and nurses, he took the co-ed into the chamber, ran up the pressure and administered 100% Oxygen by mask for two hours. Next day she was given two more treatments that lasted 90 minutes each. On her third day in the tank her fever dropped, the pain eased—and the doctor's side, the deadly disease had been halted.

On September 29th Sandra Olson went into the chamber for one final hyperbaric treatment and emerged well. It took plastic surgery to repair her abdomen with synthetic muscle. But in time she was able to return to the university—and active enough to become a campus beauty queen.

The next to be saved was, curiously, a young (36) surgeon, Dr. John H. Turgeson of Madison, Wisconsin. His car was struck at a highway intersection as he drove home on a raw night in March 1964. The crash shattered his pelvic bones, sheared the sacroiliac joint, ripped open his right hip. He was flung into a muddy field where dirty cornstalks penetrated his gaping wounds.

Rushed back to Madison General Hospital, he was carefully patched up. At first, he seemed to be doing okay. But two days later his temperature job to 105, his pulse went from 72 to 160, and he became delirious. Within hours his doctor saw grim signs—the skin around his wound turning the color of dull copper. It felt spongy, cracked audibly when touched, and smelled rotten. They pared away all the black tissue, gave Turgeson 24 units of blood, and massive shots of penicillin. But the wildfire infection refused to be checked.

Turgeson's hospital colleagues were not optimistic. Then came another of those odd little breaks that often characterize the fitful advance of hyperbaria. Dr. John Brandabur, an internist friend, recalled an article in the British medical journal Lancet about use of a tank to treat gas gangrene.

Quickly he re-read it and began phoning around to find the nearest chamber. There was a brand new complex 150 miles away in a Chicago suburb, Lutheran General Hospital in Park Ridge, Illinois.

On the National Guard plane, Turgeson stopped breathing for one minute 20 seconds by Brandabur's watch. When Turgeson was rolled into the Lutheran chamber at 9pm on Saturday, March 14th, his right thigh had swollen three times its normal size, and the discoloration had spread from knees to armpits, and was sprinkled with hideous purple blisters.

It required an hour for Dr. Otto Trippel, Lutheran staff surgeon, and Brandabur to trim away the decaying flesh. Turgeson was unconscious, so they did a myringotomy (lancing the eardrums) otherwise the tank pressure could rupture them. Conscious, he might have popped his ears himself by swallowing. The tank was pressurized and 100% oxygen was administered by face mask. Within 45 minutes the patient actually began to get well. His temperature fell to 100, his pulse slowed from 160 to 100, and he came out of his coma. The oxygen tension in his blood had risen 15 times above normal and overpowered the Clostridium perfringens.

His first treatment lasted three hours, with the final 50 minutes devoted to slowly decompressing him. He was pressurized 16 times in the next five days, and then the wounds began to heal. The crisis was over.

The Saturday Evening Post (September 19th, 1964) described his experience along with other triumphs of the then-new "miracle tanks" and quoted Turgeson: "I knew I was dying when I arrived at the hospital in Park Ridge... I really didn't think I would pull through."

After skin grafts and physical therapy treatments, Turgeson was able to resume his practice in cardiovascular surgery. Reading about him, I jumped to the conclusion that this doctor—because of such a personal close call—would be today an eager booster, making certain his own patients got full advantage of the benefits of HBO. But an interview gave me a shock.

"It is very true," Turgeson told me candidly, "that I wouldn't be alive now if I hadn't been taken to the chamber, but, well, it isn't that useful... How often do you see a case of gas gangrene?"

Many physicians are uncertain today about hyperbaric therapy, as pointed out earlier. But it was startling to hear this surgeon, who owes his own life to HBO, express deep and serious doubts about its current worth and importance.

Gas gangrene can be capricious, and mysterious. Considered the case of a healthy 38-year-old housewife suddenly developing extensive gas gangrene in a buttock and thigh. Milwaukee's Kindwall, who treated—and saved—her at St Luke's Hospital found no injury, not even a break in the skin. "The only unusual event that could be isolated in her history," Kindwall said, "was that she had been horseback riding a few days before becoming ill."

Medical science will never win every war on disease. But the hyperbaric tank unquestionably has beautifully lifted our odds against gas gangrene. Take a look at how the mortality rate has changed. Of the World War II wounded who got gas gangrene, 34% died even with good treatment, 60% if treatment was delayed, and 90 to 100% when no treatment was available.

Of 130 gas gangrene victims given hyperbaric treatment during the last 10 years at Wilhelmina Hospital in Amsterdam, only 14 died directly of the infection. 15 others succumbed during treatment, but from other specific causes such as heart attacks, pulmonary embolism, cancer, intestinal obstruction, or other infections.

This, the most thorough and extensive analysis available at this writing, appeared in the journal Surgery, Gynecology & Obstetrics (April 1972). In their summary, Drs. B. Podin, A. Groenvald and Ite Boerema of Wilhelmina Hospital pointed out:

"...the use of hyperbaric oxygen in the therapy of gas gangrene is the therapy of choice. If the condition of the patient is such that he will survive five treatments in the hyperbaric chamber, the gas gangrene will be cured.

Therefore, early diagnosis is of vital importance. The survival rate in this series was 77.7 per cent. Permanent invalidity was reduced to a minimum as no emergency amputations were performed."

9

BURNS, STROKE, CARBON MONOXIDE

Burns

A roaring explosion deep in a Japanese coal mine in 1965 is responsible for the accidental discovery that hyperbaric therapy speeds the healing of burns and reduces infection.

Many of the miners overcome by carbon dioxide were rushed to the hospital's hyperbaric chamber. A few days later the Japanese physicians noted a remarkable coincidence. The burns on the carbon monoxide patients were healing faster than those on the other burned miners. The only difference in treatment—one group had been in the tank.

Hyperbarists in the United States were quick to utilize these findings. Milwaukee's Kindwall points out that in burns the blood supply to the victim's skin is compromised due to coagulation necrosis and edema. "If the cells whose blood supply has been compromised," Kindwall explains, "can be artificially oxygenated until the circulation is reestablished, greater survival of tissue in the burned areas can be anticipated."

Some of the most extensive clinical burn research has been done at Long Beach Naval Hospital, where Hart treats even patients who formerly would have been considered hopeless and reports excellent results. Under hyperbaric treatment serious burns appear to heal twice as quickly and require fewer skin grafts.

When burn victims are brought to the tank within 24 hours of injury, Hart finds that the oxygen quickly reduces edema thus accelerating eschar formation, which is the destroyed tissue that must slough off the wound, a development that in turn decreases the patient's electrolyte and colloid demands. The new blood supply develops more rapidly and hastens the opportunity for skin grafting.

Hart's research nurse, Alice L. Gaul, described to me one of their most critical cases, a man who had 60% third-degree burns from a combination of gasoline and electricity. His camper crashed into a power pole, knocking down the high-voltage wire. He grabbed the line to throw it off his burning car and totally carbonized his arm, which had to be amputated.

His chances of surviving such an injury were about zero. What makes his case really bad was that it involved his upper trunk, with a combination of electrical and regular flame burns.

In an electrical burn, doctors can't determine where all the current has gone and what underneath tissue has been killed. Whether this patient was going to lose his neck muscles, Hart couldn't tell for quite a while. The third degree burns covered his chest, throat, entire face, his eyelids were burned off and he eventually lost one eye as well as his arm.

He was lucky though, Mrs. Gaul explains, that he didn't require a tracheostomy (insertion of a tube into the windpipe) to facilitate breathing.

"This is a damned-if-you do-and damned-if-you-don't thing in treatment of burns," she said. "Because if you put a trach through the contaminated wound the patient is much more likely to get pneumonia, and if you don't do it maybe they can't breathe."

The hyperbaric chamber reduces the edema (swelling that in this type of throat burn might cause choking) so quickly that Hart at that time had tracked only two burned patients, both of whom were extensively burned.

The camper-wreck victim recovered, had plastic surgery, and went back to his job.

Mrs. Gaul says the hyperbaric chamber also means that burn patients have much less pain, and much less psychological depression, which always accompanies a severe burn.

Stroke

Not every stroke patient will respond—especially if the cause is hemorrhagic—but many doctors feel hyperbaric treatment (if they know about it) Is at least worth a try. Some results are dramatic, such as this case:

The place was Milwaukee, January 1967. Morris Holzman, a widely known lake-resort owner, was seventy-two, blind, paralyzed on his left side, and so confused from a stroke eight months before that he thought he was in Chicago. Actually, he was being rolled into County Emergency Hospital's sturdy little hyperbaric chamber.

Twenty-four hours later "His sight had improved enough for him to see a doctor coming up the walk," reported the Milwaukee Journal. Two days later he could watch television. In another few days he got out of bed and walked with a cane.

"Before he was like a blind, babbling baby," exclaimed his son-in-law. "Just look at him now! Amazing!"

This comment touches on one of the appealing dividends when this treatment is successful. About 200,000 people die annually in the United States from strokes, but two thirds of those stricken who are under 65, and a smaller percentage of those older, survive to fill beds and long-term care facilities, or become dependent on relatives.

Some hospitals see Improvement in as few as one of six stroke patients. And doctors are unable to determine in advance just which patients will get better under HBO. Some "fresh strokes"—the response seems to be better the faster they get to a tank—walk out of the chamber after only thirty minutes of breathing oxygen at 3 ATA.

Reporting on twenty cases created at Milwaukee County Emergency Hospital's tank, End cites a 73-year-old who was having his third stroke within a year. With the first, he was confined to the hospital three weeks, and the second kept him hospitalized three months. This time the doctor decided to try hyperbaric treatment. Six hours after the third stroke, the patient was taken into the tank hemiplegic and aphasic (paralyzed on one side and unable to speak or comprehend) but conscious. He walked out of the chamber in 30 minutes and left the hospital in nine days.

Similar results are reported by physicians at a dozen other medical centers. At Saint Barnabas Medical Center, a Newark dentist who suffered a stroke went into the tank "and was up in 30 minutes dancing with the nurse."

End got good or excellent results with twelve of the first twenty consecutive stroke patients he ran through his tank, including three who are in the acute, progressive stage. The eight who showed little or no improvement included four, who In fairness, should not be counted statistically. One, 83-years-old, already was in extremis (at the point of death), two had previous chronic brain diseases, and one sixty-eight, developed transient pneumonitis and couldn't continue treatment—the only bad reaction in 200 stroke treatments. That is an improvement ratio of 3 to 1, or twelve helped and four not improved.

By quickly correcting hypoxia low oxygen tension in the body in acute strokes, End says, hyperbaric oxygen may be expected to minimize brain damage, reduce arterial spasm, encourage recovery of function, and provide time for careful diagnosis and treatment. In chronic strokes he has seen it bring marked improvement long after the initial occlusion, and thus a valuable addition to established forms of treatment.

Stroke patients are usually pressurized at 2.5 or 3 ATA for ninety minutes, during which time they breathe 100% oxygen via face mask. Most hospitals give two such treatments daily.

At Duke University Medical Center, the first experience was not very good. Reporting on twenty five stroke patients, Dr. Herbert

Saltzman said the tank immediately shot more oxygen into the brain of all. Yet twelve did not respond in the least. Eight showed dramatic immediate Improvement after five to ten minutes—being able to move their hands, talk, etc. Only two of these, however, were permanently better.

The human body has, of course, a great ability for healing itself. And most stroke patients—given enough time—will get better. Mount Sinai's Hospital's Jacobson points out that "this means there are many cells which, though they are not functioning at the time, are still alive and will eventually recover. There may be areas of the brain that can be kept alive by hyperbaric oxygenation, although the return of function is not immediately apparent. It will be necessary to treat the acutely ill patient for sustained periods probably over four or five days."

Saltzman, however, believes the problem of oxygen toxicity must be solved before "we can indulge in the higher risk of substantially prolonged therapy."

Several conditions which are similar to and sometimes confused with stroke are produced by air embolisms. Senility is another aspect of cerebral oxygen insufficiency, which has been stunningly reversed although nowhere near the "Fountain of Youth" level. The many ramifications of this will be fully discussed in chapter 11.

A third aspect of insufficiency is vertigo—for which nothing could be done until the advent of HBO. These patients show no clinical symptoms of stroke, complain of persistent disturbance of balance, gait, and coordination.

Treating several non-seniles for other reasons, Kindwall in Milwaukee made the accidental discovery that all lost their vertigo disability in the tank.

"The mechanism," said Kindwall, "is not understood. We do not know how long improvement persists, although one patient treated eight months ago still maintains her Improvement."

Carbon Monoxide

An ambulance screamed up to Saint Luke's Hospital in Milwaukee with a 40-year-old man who was decerebrate—a condition roughly equivalent to a chicken with its head cut off. Shoveling snow, he had stepped into the garage where the car was running to get warm. Now he was deeply unconscious from carbon monoxide, his arms and legs thrashing about, his brain scarcely functioning.

His blood was 80% saturated with carbon monoxide. Saturation as low as 30% can kill and 66%, if untreated, is uniformly fatal.

Kindwall took him directly into the hyperbaric chamber and started pressurizing. When the pressure reached 20 pounds per square inch, Kindwall said to the nurse: "When we get to 30 PSI, he'll be lucid."

Then a voice from under the oxygen mask said, "I'm lucid."

This unusual case illustrates the tank's dramatic effectiveness in this illness. Carbon monoxide, the product of imperfect burning, Is odorless, invisible, and slightly lighter than air. It is so deadly that air containing only 1% carbon monoxide can snuff out life in 10 minutes.

Carbon monoxide kills by asphyxiation, blocking delivery of oxygen to vital tissues, of which the brain is the most vulnerable. Oxygen, of course, normally is transported to the tissues by the hemoglobin in the red blood cells. But hemoglobin is about 250 times more attracted to carbon monoxide than to oxygen; thus, any of this poison gas inhaled zooms on a sort of top priority into the bloodstream, brushing oxygen aside.

If the victim is taken out into fresh air it takes five hours, 20 minutes—provided he's breathing—before half the carbon monoxide is eliminated from his blood. Meanwhile he may die or suffer permanent brain damage. If the ambulance driver or intern gives a hundred percent oxygen by mask, the washout time —as it is called—will be cut to 1 hour 20 minutes.

But in a tank at 3 ATA and breathing 100% oxygen, the washout time is only 23 minutes! Also, the risk of brain damage drops drastically because the pressurization both reduces brain swelling and sends extra oxygen to the brain via the plasma.

Medical centers with tanks in all parts of the country have heartening statistics on salvage of would-be suicides who stuck their heads in the gas oven or left the car motor running in a closed garage, as well as for victims of accidental smoke and exhaust inhalation.

In a recent single year in Milwaukee, Saint Luke's hyperbaric chambers treated fifty-nine carbon monoxide victims. Of those patients who reached the hospital alive, there was only one monoxide fatality —child who first has been taken elsewhere, causing a three-hour delay in treatment.

Smoke inhalation victims usually suffer also some carbon monoxide poisoning, but even those who do not will benefit from hyperbaric treatment because the tank steps up their sagging oxygen tension and at the same time reduces edema in the lungs.

Experts realize that countless thousands of fire victims have died not because of burns but through failure to receive treatment for carbon monoxide poisoning. Such deaths obviously can become fewer when more fireman and ambulance drivers are alerted to the HBO potential. Dr. Bashir A. Zikria of Columbia University's College of Physicians and Surgeons made the situation clear in a review of a series of autopsies. Of 105 fire victims with less than 40% of the body surface burned, he found 77% should have survived, and 76% of these fatalities were related to respiratory complications, such as carbon monoxide or smoke poisoning.

Hyperbaric treatment also is recommended for cyanide poisoning. In Canada a man trying to elude police slipped into an electroplating factory and hid in a vat of what looked to be dirty water. It was a deadly poison—Cyanide and sodium hydroxide solution. He was found unconscious, fished out, hosed down, and rushed to the hospital. He was at once put into the hyperbaric chamber at 3 ATA with 100% oxygen administered by mask.

Just in the nick of time, too. Dr. W. G. Trapp, reporting the case in the Canadian Medical Association journal in 1970, said the fugitive awoke within an hour and had an uneventful recovery.

Air Embolism

An air bubble loose in the bloodstream is big trouble. If it is detected soon enough, the hyperbaric chamber usually can handle it.

Technical errors during open heart surgery can cause an air embolism. Or a scuba diver ascending too abruptly may get one from rupturing a lung sac. The bubble often blocks blood flow to the brain. The victim goes into a coma, is paralyzed, half-blind, and possibly seized by convulsions.

Doctors must somehow squeeze out the air bubble before anoxia damages the brain or causes death. The best treatment is to use heavy pressure in the tank. At 6 ATA the compressive effect gradually shrinks the bubble to 1/6 its initial size. Such a reduction may permit the bubble to move on, unblocking the blood circulation, and give the human physiology an opportunity in the next day or two to reabsorb or expel the offending air pocket.

Even freak accidents cause these bubbles. A 16-year-old girl practicing mouth to mouth Yoga breathing with her boyfriend fell over unconscious. She was dead on arrival at the emergency room. The autopsy revealed air in her heart and the carotid arteries. She obviously had over strained and ruptured her lungs.

More fortunate was a woman, 23, undergoing surgery for insertion of an artificial heart valve. When the surgeon stuck the cannula into her aorta, air slipped into the blood vessel. A few hours later she came out of the anesthesia paralyzed and half blind. She was rushed to the tank at Veterans Administration Hospital at Buffalo,

New York, arriving six and a half hours after the accident. Alvis tried compressing her at 2.8 ATA for thirty minutes. She was given 100% oxygen by mask. But there was no change.

Then Alvis knew he had to shoot the works if there was any chance to save the woman. This means committing the patient and one doctor and a technician to a grueling 38-hour stay inside the tank. The pressure is rapidly increased to 6 ATA—equivalent to diving 165 feet beneath the sea—and held there for two hours. Then it is lowered in accordance with gradual steps set out in the US Navy Diver decompression table. It takes a day and a half to get back to a 1 ATA, sea level.

Because tension and fatigue may affect judgment of the medical personnel inside the chamber, the physician on duty outside—in this case Alvis—makes the decisions.

In about two hours the woman began to get feeling back in her side. After twenty-eight hours she could move her arm, and later her leg. Eight hours after getting out of the tank her sight returned to normal. And twenty-five days after the operation she luckily was able to leave the Buffalo Hospital—with no indication of brain damage.

Experts believe many unexplained cerebral accidents are undiagnosed air bubbles—and in most cases, unfortunately, HBO is not even called on for help. Alvis said in The Journal of the American Medical Association:

... Considering the likelihood that occult air embolism has been more common than usually thought, we suggest that hyperbaric therapy should be used when there are significant neurological dysfunction immediately after open heart surgery.

Weightlifters and others trying to breathe under strain may rupture their lung lining and induce air emboli. Many women have attempted self-abortion by inserting a catheter into the uterus without realizing that this can easily rupture the vascular bed and force an air bubble into the circulatory system.

Four such cases were cited by French physicians on the staff of the Raymond Poincaré Hospital in Paris before the conference at Duke University in 1965. Treated at 2 ATA for four or five days, two of the women recovered. One, twenty-six, escaped unmarred. But the other survivor, thirty-six, had some brain damage, including impaired vision.

Most medical authorities believe heavy pressure, applied in a hyperbaric chamber as rapidly as possible, is essential for complete recovery from air embolism.

The point was emphasized at the Duke Conference by one of the leading American hyperbaric authorities, Lanphier of Buffalo.

Commenting on the Paris case, he said:

"If I got hold of an early air embolism, I would want to compress the bubble and get prompt relief of the symptoms. And if it's my brain and somebody puts me on oxygen at 2 atmospheres and then sits down and watches my EEG waiting for something to happen, if I pull through, he won't!"

Other Applications

Hyperbaric therapy has been found beneficial in about a dozen other disease and injury-oriented conditions. The list (not necessarily in order of importance):

Traumatic head injury, which invariably produces cerebral edema further compounding the insult to the brain as expansion within the skulls squeezes off the blood supply. HBO immediately decreases pressure 40 to 50 percent—at 3 ATA the brain will shrink two inches! —while at the same time providing an extra inflow of oxygen.

Drowning, Asphyxia, or Electrocution—in which the benefit also is reduction of cerebral edema.

Skin grafts, which are essentially anoxic for two or three days until the capillaries can invade the graft and reestablish blood circulation.

Skin ulcers, including the chronic undermining type (Meleney), as well as most which result from diabetes. Meleney ulcers may heal permanently because the infection is overcome. Diabetic ulcers usually occur because of changes in the small peripheral blood vessels and resultant poor tissue oxygenation. These ulcers may heal, and HBO may promote healing but there is no evidence of basic change in the underlying causes. These ulcers have a high recurrence rate probability, one expert warns.

Tetanus, an essentially anaerobic infection known as lockjaw. Astoundingly successful case histories have been reported by some therapists, but others have found results disappointing.

Syphilis, mentioned here because of the recent tendency of the infection to become more immune to penicillin, except in massive doses; an anaerobic infection that was cured as early as 1918 in the first US hyperbaric chamber.

Sickle cell anemia crisis, a hereditary trait principally among the Negro race, and which HBO promptly reverses, although there is no known cure.

Decompression sickness, the "bends" suffered by caisson workers, professional and scuba divers who ascend too quickly from a prolonged stay below the thirty-three foot depth, trapping nitrogen bubbles in their tissues.

Blood loss anemia, exceedingly dangerous when suffered by members of religious cults (such as Jehovah's Witness) whose belief forbids blood transfusion.

Pulmonary insufficiency, such as pneumonia.

Actinomycosis, a rare but difficult infection caused by fungus.

Some hyperbaric chamber therapists also indicate benefit in treatment of gastric ulcer and intestinal obstructions. The theory in intestinal obstructions is that the tank has a compressive effect on this condition, which in most hospitals has a 20 to 25 percent mortality.

However, one expert points out that the treatment of intestinal obstruction is surgical and that compressing the gas and the bowel may facilitate operation slightly. But this is not often of significant content. He also takes the view that the evidence to support HBO's usefulness in gastric ulcer is presently too flimsy to warrant listing.

10

IN THE V.I.P. SPOTLIGHT

At mid-afternoon on December 5th, 1968, the sleek limousine from New York whirled up to the side entrance of Saint Barnabas Medical Center. The chauffeur sprang out to open doors. Jacqueline Kennedy Onassis, in a light raincoat and dark glasses, emerged with easy grace. She smiled at the reporters but said nothing and was immediately ushered inside. Aristotle Onassis, swarthy, dark-suited, solemn and equally uncommunicative, followed. They were trailed into the hospital by the limousine's third passenger, his bright-eyed daughter Christina.

Jackie's fabulous $20,000,000 honeymoon was in full swing. Just forty-seven days earlier she had married the Greek shipping multi-millionaire.

Their visit to the Saint Barnabas hyperbaric chamber smelled like good copy to the reporters. The Newark papers and the AP and UPI were covering. The movie magazines also were represented. The Hollywood editors literally pounced on the event. For years on any pretext, they had clutched the doe-eyed First Lady's willowy figure to their covers to fill the Marilyn Monroe void. And so now, their writers dutifully trumpeted the Saint Barnabas dive in extravagant headlines trying to satiate the celebrity-itis hunger of yearning housewives lulling away afternoon tedium under beauty shop dryers from Maine to California.

If these readers got a vicarious thrill, it was undeserved. To Jackie the dive was just a lark. And it meant very little to Ari.

Their seventy-five mile round trip from Manhattan to the Livingston, New Jersey Medical Center leaves no significant mark on the modern history of hyperbaric medicine. It is at most a colorful footnote indicative of the decade of intermittent publicity that heralded the emergence in the 1960s of the bevy of big and expensive hyperbaric chambers in America.

As one after another of these great tanks went into service, frequent "miracle" healings were chronicled by the newspapers, radio, TV and weekly news magazines, critically examined and debated in the medical journals, and enthusiastically marveled at by scores of periodicals ranging from Saturday Evening post and Readers Digest to Popular Mechanics and Fire Engineering.

It had been Ari's curiosity, not Jackie's, that brought them to Saint Barnabas this December afternoon. Ari, as reporters learned later, wanted to see firsthand what the tank looked like, how it worked, what a patient would experience.

His interest had been stirred six months previously by a long-time friend, the American aluminum tycoon J. Lewis Reynolds of Richmond, Virginia. Talking other business, Reynolds had remarked that his company's efforts to develop a new deep-diving submarine was leading him into a study of pressure physiology.

"I stumbled onto something that is utterly fascinating," Reynolds said. "Hyperbaric medicine."

Reynolds had seen in this a therapeutic potential that literally inflamed his imagination. He hit on an idea to improve the lives of older people, especially those showing signs of senility.

He intended to build a large apartment complex in Richmond that would have its own hyperbaric chamber, and the residents could not only live in the pressurized environment but work in it as well.

He wanted the biggest tank in the world with room enough for 1,000 people.

The scheme definitely intrigued Onassis. So much so that although he was honeymooning when Reynolds finally invited him to sample a dive in the hyperbaric chamber at Saint Barnabas, Onassis readily agreed to go along. Jackie, too, thought it would be interesting.

Their host and guide was Anthony Scala, president of Saint Barnabas Medical Center, and probably America's most dynamic HBO "salesman." The hospital had become virtually his whole life, and he was fascinated by the success and potential of hyperbaric medicine. Scala, son of a glass blower, struggled for an education, worked in a factory laboratory and developed the tubing that paved the way for the fluorescent lamp. He parlayed this break into a multi-million dollar electronics manufacturing concern which in the 50s he sold to Tung-Sol Electric. In "retirement" he unleashed his energy and Imagination on the task of moving Saint Barnabas out of Newark's slums into the suburbs where it could be revitalized as a modern 650-bed Hospital

Proud, knowledgeable, and articulate, Scala escorted the Onassis-Reynolds VIP party to the hyperbaric wing. Jackie may have expected to encounter some awkward, clanking, boiler-like contraption. If so, entering the control room gave her a surprise. It was a quiet, pleasant, orderly room in fresh pastel colors.

Head Nurse Bob Cornish sat at a huge L-shaped control panel, the most prominent visible feature of the room. Six feet high and about fifteen feet long, the board was covered with about one hundred dials, gauges, switches, and knobs that regulate the atmosphere in the six locks in the Twin Chambers. Scala pointed out to his visitors that Cornish could observe on TV screens on his panel whatever was happening inside the tanks, just one safety precaution.

With the heavy doors standing open, Jackie looked all the way through the 45-foot tanks. Most people compare a hyperbaric chamber interior to how they imagine it looks inside a large submarine. The sides were curved, of course, with heavy portholes in these walls. The chamber was floored with a series of metal plates, affording space for about twenty patients to sit in regular office-type chairs, or in wheelchairs. Patients could also be rolled in on beds.

Narrow grills along the edge of the floor and larger ones in the ceiling permitted circulation of air within the hull. Oxygen masks dangled from hoses attached along the walls, and large operating room lights were suspended from the ceiling; music was piped in. The colors harmonized with the pleasant décor of the adjacent rooms.

These tanks had been set in place during construction of the building so that all floors were flush, with no climbing up or down necessary to enter the chamber. The doors were heavy, thick, but wide and tall and marvelously balanced. They closed noiselessly at finger touch.

Scala introduced Jackie and the others to his chief operator, Stew Beakley, a handsome, fortyish retired Canadian Navy diver. Beakley explained that all watches, hearing aids, pens, cigarettes, matches and lighters would be left outside the chamber; the crystal would pop right out of a watch.

Once they were inside and the tank "buttoned up," the pressure was raised slowly. Compressed air goes in through a silencer, resulting in a noise level about equal to that of a small business office.

They would be in the chamber no longer than an hour on this sample dive.

The pressure had been building up barely two minutes when Jackie felt ear pain. Beakley saw her wince and promptly stopped the pressurization. He showed her how to make her ears pop to relieve the pressure. If an unconscious patient is taken into the chamber usually a myringotomy is performed; the eardrums are lanced with a surgical needle, otherwise the pressure might rupture the tympanic membrane.

As the pressure increased to three ATA, the VIPs felt a slight increase in the air temperature of the chamber due to the adiabatic heat of compression. But this was minimized by cooling coils located beneath the floor plates.

No one experienced any strange physical sensations, though they kept swallowing at intervals or doing the Valsalva maneuver to keep their inner ear pressure balanced, and some felt twinges of ear pain if they were too slow making their ears pop. Scala walked about demonstrating how to hold the soft rubber face mask tight against nose and mouth so his guests could be ready to breathe pure oxygen when they reach full pressurization.

After about seven or eight minutes, Beakley saw that they had reached a pressure of about 2.5 ATA.

Beakley turned and spoke to Jackie. "Who do I sound like?"

She started in surprise, and then smiled brightly. "Like Donald Duck!"

"You do, too!" Beakley gave a friendly laugh. "We all sound that way. The pressure causes it. The increased density of the air. Don't try to whistle—you can't."

Scala indicated it was time to begin breathing oxygen through their face masks. This was simple and pleasant. Most of them sat in chairs. Onassis intermittently walked about closely examining the chamber. He queried Scala about a number of technical matters, indicating he had an above average understanding of the principles of pressurization.

After an hour and a quarter Beakley signaled Cornish to begin decompression, a process in which the air is gradually bled out of the chamber. There was no hissing sound because of the silencers on the air lines, but there was a slight cooling effect due to expansion of the air. Heating coils under the floor were triggered by thermostats to automatically compensate for this chill.

Another 10 minutes and Beakley swung open the doors. They were now back at sea level pressure. Jackie and the others emerged, feeling lightheaded for a few minutes. Then they got the characteristic aftereffect of a dive—a solid sense of well-being.

Ari wanted to see the machinery. Scala led him to the basement. Onassis studied compressors, valving arrangements, reserve holding tanks for air, the emergency supply—a battery of individual compressed air cylinders. Then Onassis collected his new bride, his daughter, and whisked away in the limousine.

Reynolds stayed behind and held a press conference at the hospital to let the world in on his apartment scheme.

Possibly without realizing it, Reynolds had been bitten by the same grandiose ambition which inspired Dr Cunningham and Timken. But Reynolds was thinking bigger—his idea was to construct a tank probably ten or fifteen times as large as the previous world's largest, the steel ball in Cleveland.

Reynolds impressed the reporters; to them he looked like a man in a hurry. He vowed he would get his engineers in Richmond busy that very weekend on the plans. And Saint Barnabas would be asked to operate the apartment complex.

Costs hadn't yet been calculated, but Reynolds was so optimistic he announced the site for his second hyperbaric apartment complex. It would be on a former Navy base he had purchased at Jacksonville, Florida.

Unfortunately, it didn't work out. This scheme never got much beyond talk. Reynolds did not build the apartment complex in Richmond. And if his engineers ever actually designed the 1000 person tank, it was not made public. He did nothing at Jacksonville.

This was not at all surprising. Actually, it was further attestation to the difficulty of getting broad-based support in business and medical circles for such enterprises. Also, a 1000 person chamber faced formidable cost in design barriers.

Even so, such dreams die hard. Reynolds—as late as June 1972—still clung to his. He had not yet abandoned the idea. He still wanted to go ahead, according to associates in the executive suite at Richmond, but had not "because of business conditions." It seems unlikely the scheme was greeted with enthusiasm by other directors of the vast Reynolds company. Louis Reynolds' spokesman, giving me a fill-in on the status of his project, pointedly explained; "When he does this, it will be a personal undertaking, not a Reynolds company project."

Ari Onassis— who is in his 60s is so fit, according to Louis Reynolds, that he swims two miles a day—gave no public hint of further interest in hyperbaric therapy.

Reynolds undoubtedly was ahead of his time. But he was on solid ground in his concept that HBO can markedly benefit and brighten the life of senior citizens who are losing their cognitive powers.

My investigation indicates use of hyperbaric chambers may present a tremendous untapped resource for business. Someday the "executive brush-up" maybe come as routine as vacations.

The case of a prominent Dallas, Texas, industrialist is a classic example of how HBO can restore an aging executive.

Major William F. Long got into aviation as a 22-year-old World War I pilot. He had guts and brass; for a 1921 Galveston Air Show he set a plane afire and bailed out, earning$ 4,000 for the stunt. Later he sold planes, opened a big flying school, had aircraft maintenance shops in Dallas, and in 1943 founded Pioneer Airlines (which merged with Continental in 1954). He had a busy and active fifty years as a business executive, but in 1970—at age 75—he found himself forgetful and weak; so, he decided to give up control of his vast enterprises.

Fortunately, just then, he heard how hyperbaric treatments can counteract the dark side of growing old.

He arrived at Saint Barnabas in a wheelchair. He checked into the hospital, and doctors there gave him two 90-minute dives daily. Within three or four days he had perked up; and at the end of two weeks felt better than he had in years.

Elated that his memory and vigor had been restored, Major Long flew back to Dallas and took charge of his business again. Doctors warned that the rejuvenative effects usually are transitory. Major Long had a simple remedy for that. When the new mental stimulus began to wear off, he went back to Saint Barnabas for another series of dives—the "brush-up." In his case these were necessary every four to six months.

Another who swears by the mental stimulus derived from HBO is the noted Kentucky politician-lawyer John Young Brown, Sr., of Lexington and Louisville.

It was Brown who first told me about HBO. We ran into each other in the fall of 1971 at a reception Kentucky Governor Louis Nunn gave in the Mansion to celebrate publication of a new pictorial history of the Commonwealth. I knew Brown to be about 70—and yet the distinguished fellow I could see across the ballroom examining the new book looked about 40. Could that be John Y., Sr.? I hadn't seen him since his last political race two or three years before, I went over—and it was John Y. As we chatted, he suddenly was telling me about his own discovery of HBO, which came directly because of a bitter personal tragedy.

In September 1970 his daughter Pamela, a model and actress, was lost over the Atlantic while trying to fly a balloon from Long Island to France. After a long, futile aerial search, Brown was exhausted physically and mentally. He knew Onassis and Senator Everett McKinley Dirksen had been to Saint Barnabas. Brown went, and recalls:

"I was able to stay only three days, and it took six dives. It helped me tremendously. My mind cleared up. I could remember names again. I could think straight, I felt better. Even my eyesight improved; I didn't need reading glasses. Later I went back for a longer course. And I go every so often for a brush-up. It is a marvelous thing.

Brown has recruited many HBO converts. He took his wife to the same Barnabas tank because she has hepatitis—which normally would not be affected by oxygenation—but she did feel better, he said, and her appetite improved so much that she was able to eat again and gain weight, and thus became stronger.

Brown also introduced Colonel Harland Sanders, the Kentucky Fried Chicken king, to the new" brush-up." Sanders, over 80 years old, said he felt new pep and vigor. The Colonel took refresher dives several times. He became so sharp and alert, in fact, that the Veterans Administration invited him to Washington, DC, to relate his experience to a conference on aging. Brown and his lawyer son, John Y. Jr., had "discovered" Sanders two decades before and provided the business guidance that made him a millionaire world personality.

Senator Dirksen spent a week at Saint Barnabas in November 1968 taking hyperbaric therapy. He suffered from emphysema. He was much impressed with the relief the dives seemed to give him.

His widow, Luella, told me in 1972: "I think he came home quite refreshed from the treatment, but according to the doctors it was not extended long enough to produce any lasting effects. I think had his work not been so pressing at the time, he might have gone back for a prolonged treatment."

Dirksen never found the time to go back. He died on September7th, 1969, at age 73.

Another emphysema victim who sought help from the Saint Barnabas chamber was Jackie Onassis' stepfather. In December 1968 when he was seventy-one years old, Hugh D. Auchincloss, a Washington, DC investment broker, was a patient for a brief time.

For the rich and famous to be fascinated by the hyperbaric chamber is neither new nor recent.

Merre Shane, who was Dr. Cunningham's nurse back in the 20s, recalls that U.S. Grant, Jr., the son of President Ulysses S Grant, was a patient in the Kansas City Sanitarium

"He was very interesting and charming, about seventy-five, as I remember," Miss Shane told me. He was owner of the US Grand Hotel in San Diego. He was a diabetic. One day he was sitting in a rocker on the porch, smoking a long-stemmed cherry meerschaum pipe, with the bowl on his knee. I asked where he got such an unusual pipe. 'It was my father's,' he said, 'when he was President.' And I said, 'Is it all intact?' He said, 'No, the Indian head is missing. When my father was out inspecting the Army, a sniper shot it off.'"

After a long period of treatment, Grant, Jr., returned to California and died in 1929 at age seventy-seven.

11

THE TANK VS. OLD AGE

Anyone who has helplessly watched the cruel fingers of senility reach out to squeeze the brain of an elderly friend or relative and leave him doddering and befuddled can easily imagine what it would mean for the hyperbaric chamber to come to the rescue as a sort of Fountain of Youth.

The minds of ten million Americans currently are being crippled by age. Any process offering revitalizing "brain food" would be a boon of incalculable worth. Not only for its humanitarianism, but also for its potential economic impact in eliminating the custodial and nursing care these oldsters now require.

Fortunately, HBO has been found effective against senility. No one should get his hopes high too quickly, because there is but a small beginning. Research is of recent origin and has raised perhaps as many intriguing new questions as it has answered. On the other hand, this specific physiologic inquiry also has started medical investigators hammering hard against the locked door of life's very mysterious room —the one wherein is hidden the baffling secret of just what does cause aging.

Oxygen plays an indisputable key role in our aging process. No one as yet has the total picture of how or why. Scientists are fiddling with a half-dozen intriguing theories, but so far, their efforts have not succeeded in extending the average lifespan in the US more than a year or two beyond the Biblical three score and 10.

The latest research is not pinned on a hope that the hyperbaric chamber specifically will lengthen our lifespan, but rather that it will enable the aged to remain alert and useful to the end of their days.

Potential value of such a medical breakthrough is reflected in population statistics; now 23 million Americans are over 65 years of age, and by the year 2000 the figure will be 28 million. Although we do not live much longer than we did in 1900, more of us reach old age. 4,000 turn 65 daily in this country, of whom 1,000 survived to swell the elderly ranks. The United States had in 1970 about 15,000 residents who were 100 years old, three times the number of centenarians in the 1950s.

The principal cause of senility is arteriosclerosis, hardening of the arteries. This disease narrows vessels carrying blood to the brain, thus diminishing its oxygen supply. The brain, gradually starved of this essential, deteriorates little by little, very slowly. Its size shrinks, some tissue actually dies, and a vast number of other cells slow down, more or less shifting into idleness and ceasing to function effectively.

A major breakdown frequently occurs in the memory mechanism. Deprived of adequate oxygen, brain cells seem to emulate the lazy laborer who just leans on a shovel and does nothing. Such weakened cells stop accepting and processing information. That means that recent memory is quickly shot, typified by inability to remember what was eaten for breakfast. Yet the cells, presumably the same cells, preserve memories of information processed long ago, such as perhaps how the sunset looked on a trip out west in 1910, or the words of a popular song in 1930.

Scientists don't believe they can do much about stepping up blood flow to the brain of elderly arteriosclerotics, because the muscle walls of their arteries have lost ability to relax and expand. But even in such reduced circulation they say HBO enriches the oxygen content and thus enables idle brain cells to again start functioning.

Experiments are underway in half a dozen US HBO centers into treatment to alleviate, or even prevent, senility. These studies were inspired by the success of one research project with a strange, oddball history. It was buried for 13 years, revived by chance, but then stalled for a couple more years, finally getting off the ground only through odd circumstances.

The heroine of this scientific melodrama is a distinguished clinical psychologist on the staff of Veterans Administration Hospital at Buffalo, New York, Eleanor Jacobs, Ph.D.

Back in 1952 she was an eager, bright-eyed brunette, interning at the Buffalo VA hospital as a clinical psychologist, and also studying for her doctorate. Her decision to become a psychologist had been inspired by two years (1944-46) spent in the WAVES as a Navy Hospital Corpsman. After discharge from the Navy, she studied under the GI bill.

In turn Jacobs worked in a psychiatric ward and assisted a research physician carrying out a curious experiment; he was attempting to lessen acute anxiety in some patients by causing them to periodically inhale carbon dioxide. Three or four were assigned to her for individual psychotherapy,

The improvement in her patients was impressive. She was "amazed" that things they had been able to remember, facts that were blocked out of memory, were so much more readily available after they had inhaled carbon dioxide.

She had always wanted to work in memory and discussed it with the researcher. He cautioned her not to jump to conclusions. The patients were breathing what he termed a "very interesting" combination—30% carbon dioxide and 70% pure oxygen. Did she know whether she was interested in the effect of the carbon dioxide, or of the oxygen?

Jacobs realized she wasn't sure. She did a lot of reading and came up with the notion she was interested in the effects of oxygen. She prepared a research protocol, to study not aged but younger patients. She proposed to try to determine whether learning something new while in an atmosphere of elevated levels of oxygen would result in better retention of the material.

The hospital's research committee told her she was "terribly naïve". They told her there was no known way of measuring the amount of oxygen that would actually get into the bloodstream and tissue. Besides it would be a project for a physician, not a psychologist; she could just forget it.

Eleanor Jacobs thought her superiors knew what they were talking about; dutifully she stuck the idea in her file and forgot all about it. Her full attention turned to becoming a good clinical psychologist, interested in diagnostic testing and organic brain damage.

Something happened in 1965 to revive her interest in oxygen experimentation. The Buffalo Veterans Hospital got a hyperbaric chamber.

Talk across the country of the tanks help in open heart surgery had piqued the interest of two of the VA hospitals surgeons, Drs. Andrew Gage and William Chardack. They put in a request for a hyperbaric chamber for research work and the VA officials in Washington listened, with good reason. Gage and Chardack had already given considerable luster to the VA Medical image by developing in 1960 an implanted battery-operated pacemaker to stimulate a regular heartbeat. Subsequently Gage and Chardack became disenchanted with surgery in the tank.

But from the beginning of its installation in Buffalo, Jacobs, administrator then of a psychiatric ward, was intrigued by this new research tool. She remembered the discarded 1952 project and mentioned to Bernie Reed, the hospital's management analyst, that she would like to exhume it.

One day Reed brought to her office the veteran former Navy physician who had come to Buffalo in 1964 to direct the Hyperbaric medicine Department, Harry J. Alvis. He was the first staff physician who didn't discourage her; but he did point out there were plenty of reasons why her idea wouldn't work; but he also said nobody had ever tried it either. Alvis urged her to read up on hyperbaric medicine and they might try the experiment.

But desire and good intentions were not enough. As ward administrator, Jacobs was tied to a 12-hour shift seven days a week. The hospital wouldn't give her any time for research. No replacement was available to spring her from the Ward. She fussed and fumed. That did no good; and the impasse dragged on two years.

By the fall of 1967 Jacobs was so fed up she forced a showdown. Fortunately, she won, and the upshot was that she was given half her time to spend on the oxygen research project.

Others were also interested in this research. Both Alvis and Jacobs were teaching at State University of New York at Buffalo, whose School of Medicine is affiliated with the VA hospital. Dr. S. Mouchly Small, professor and chairman of the Department of Psychiatry, had speculated on possible recovery of mental ability in the senile by relieving their presumed arteriosclerotic cerebral hypoxia. And Dr. Peter M. Winter of the school had a strong interest in oxygen toxicity.

The four joined forces, but this team of researchers was ready to begin long before formal approval emerged from the slow grinding of the wheels of bureaucracy. It was not until February 1968 that Jacobs was cleared to put the first experimental patients in the hyperbaric chamber.

Setting up their plan, the researchers saw clearly why nobody had ever attempted this experiment; it was illogical, for two reasons.

The first had to do with the autoregulatory system in human metabolism. These intricate mechanisms control the vital functions which create man's internal environment, such as oxygen use, body temperature, acid-base balance, water, and nutrient supplies including salts, fat, and sugar.

For proper respiration, the auto regulator is geared to normal air, which contains about 21% oxygen. If the inhaled air suddenly has a heavier oxygen content, the brain detects this and sends a warning to the auto regulator: Danger! Too much oxygen coming in! It can be poisonous! Do something—quick!

In response to this physiological distress call, the body does the most immediate thing it can to diminish this influx of oxygen. It cuts down on the blood flow, and hence transports less oxygen to the tissues. This is accomplished by the auto regulator telegraphing the arteries to constrict, to squeeze down, and get smaller in diameter; and by slowing the heartbeat.

Researchers considered that well-documented, medical textbook stuff, and it said clearly that the Jacobs experiment would get no place. The problem with elderly arteriosclerotics was due to already insufficient blood flow to the brain; wouldn't the higher oxygen tension just cause the cerebral arteries to clamp down even more?

Elvis and Jacob saw one flaw in the textbook premise. All the documented evidence had been based on intact cardiovascular systems in healthy young people.

To Jacobs that raised a very significant question; that it is quite possible elderly arteriosclerotic individuals do not have intact autoregulatory systems and that their vessels do not contract to the same extent or expand as they should, but the autoregulatory system may be defective and therefore the oxygen environment would not be of harm to them.

Because of another well-known fact it seemed somewhat absurd to even consider the experiment. There is no argument that cortical tissue such as the brain's gray matter is extremely dependent on oxygen and once these cells are dead, they can never be revived.

Yet Alvis and Jacobs, agreeing they didn't hope to revive dead cells, thought it worth considering that in addition to these dead cells there are perhaps a number of marginally hypoxic cells that get just enough oxygen to remain alive, but not enough to function.

If with the hyperbaric tank they could get the additional oxygen and nutrients to those marginally hypoxic, functionally ineffective cells, might not the idle cells recoup their power to act?

With little more than her maverick idea and a high-pressure tank she as yet knew little about, Eleanor Jacobs was ready to plunge into a vast uncharted physiologic wilderness.

Her aim was to improve short-term memory and mentally deteriorated oldsters; but how is that created? Psychology textbooks describe a memory trace, or engram; but nobody has ever seen one. There are also two rivalries on how memory is established—by consolidation or transfer.

In the face of this and other mysteries of man's physiology, Jacobs and Alvis were really in the dark on precisely how to use the hyperbaric chamber in this study. How much oxygen should they give? At what pressure? What should be the duration of each dive? And for how many days?

Based on his Navy experience with oxygen under pressure, Alvis believed relatively equal exposures with equal time between exposures would constitute a good program. He also worked on the notion that the old people being tested ought to receive maximum oxygen pickup with minimum toxicity hazard.

Jacobs and Alvis decided to pressurize their elderly arteriosclerotics in the safest range—2.5 ATA—for ninety minutes, each morning and each afternoon, for fifteen consecutive days. The subjects would breathe 100% Oxygen by mask.

Jacobs, incidentally, is amused that subsequent senility research elsewhere was based on a fifteen-day series, as though that time span had great scientific merit. "We had to start someplace," she says. "Fifteen days was just our ad hoc, stupid, arbitrary choice. Yet people think it's a holy cow. It isn't."

Next step was to select for the experiment subjects who, in the terms of the research protocol, "exhibited clinical manifestations of intellectual deterioration"—meaning those who had displayed a loss of recent memory, an inability to care for themselves, and a lack of interest in their surroundings. There were many such men, sixty to eighty years old, who had been in the hospital wards for months or years because of severe general deterioration due to the chronic brain syndrome associated with cerebral arteriosclerosis.

The human guinea pigs were chosen more or less at random; they were volunteers, and what is known as "informed consent"—meaning all the risks involved are clearly explained—was obtained from each, or his guardian. Their past medical records were examined, and Alvis also gave each a new physical to eliminate anyone whose cardiac, metabolic, or respiratory status would present a "calculated health risk on exposure to hyperbaric oxygenation procedures."

Jacobs selected three-seventy-year old men to be the first trial subjects and wheeled them downstairs to show them the 8 by 25-foot iron chamber and explain everything. It is a slightly awkward tank to enter, in contrast to the large walk-in tanks in use elsewhere. Entry to the Buffalo tank is via a five-foot diameter circular hatch at one end, and patients climb two steps to get over the sill. But nothing about the tank in which they would be spending three hours a day seem to faze the three men.

Before embarking on the treatments, Jacobs gave the three men a battery of psychological tests designed to measure short-term memory and conceptualization. One test gauged their ability to quickly recite the alphabet backward, another their skill in drawing diagrams they had been shown. These were standards—the Wechsler Memory Scale, the Bender-Gestalt test, and Tien's Organic Integrity test.

With these scores recorded as a basis for comparison, the three men were pressurized at 2.5 ATA for 90 minutes, twice a day for fifteen days. They experienced no untoward effects. Jacobs promptly retested them. Checking the before and after scores she felt stunned. All had shown tremendous Improvement.

She decided there was only one word for the change—"remarkable!" There was a four-fold improvement in some scores. And these were old hospital cast-offs, who had been literally out of touch for months.

The scores were so much higher, in fact, that Alvis and Jacobs feared their experiment might have slipped up. They sat down for a candid analysis, deliberately challenging its validity. What might have fouled up their protocol? First, they decided, what about just the plain attention factor? They had taken elderly, confused men, who had been content to merely sit in a geriatric ward and stare at four walls and had abruptly introduced them to a "glamorous, exciting environment"—even though it was only the tank. Could that alone have made them more alert?

Had the higher levels of oxygen, or merely the pressure of the tank, produced the improved mentation? Or had the subjects, lonely old men, tried harder on the second test because of friendly feeling toward the psychologist, a lively female? Or was there tester bias; had Jacobs unconsciously shaded the post treatment scores?

The next ten patients would be treated in pairs, under similar conditions and the paired subjects tested together. The difference would be that while in the chamber one would inhale 100% oxygen; the other would get 10% oxygen plus 90% nitrogen—a mixture that, because of the chamber's pressure, gave him about the same level of oxygen he would breathe in the ward. In other words, just normal room air.

The technicians running the chamber were instructed to rearrange and mix up the rubber hoses leading to the face masks so that neither the patients nor the psychologists testing them would know what anyone was breathing. Nor were the ward staffers to be informed there was any difference in the treatment administered.

Blood samples were being taken, one each while the patient breathed first air and then 100% oxygen outside the chamber, and four at twenty-minute intervals during treatment in the tank. These were analyzed for acid-base balance and the levels of oxygen and carbon dioxide tension. The results of the blood analysis would be kept secret from the psychologist until all comparative scoring was finished.

But even while setting up to test the five pairs of guinea pigs, Alvis and Jacobs got unexpected and startling news from the wards about the first experimental subjects.

Nurses complained that all three of the old men had become worse! Some nurses asked Jacobs to stop whatever she was doing; the patients were fine until put in the hyperbaric tank and since had become terrible.

Jacobs was both distressed and perplexed. How could an old man be getting so much more alert and showing Improvement on psychological tests, and yet change into a terrible patient?

Then suddenly she understood. For most nurses what constitutes a good geriatric patient is one who's docile, meekly accepts all orders such as to get up, go to the toilet, eat, go to bed. Pliable, almost a vegetable—in short, a good geriatric patient. One who expresses his independence and raises a little hell is not what the nurses want.

One of the patients who had so abruptly changed had been an addictive, careless smoker, always setting things on fire. His doctor had rationed him to one cigarette an hour. If nurses were busy when he came to their station to get his hourly cigarette, they might fluff him off by telling him he'd already had it. Old Charley would retreat and meekly wait.

After about 10 days of HBO, this was not the same Charley. If the nurse tried to shoo him away from her station, Charley would protest. "Don't lie to me! I had my last cigarette at ten past nine. You can see by the clock it is now five to eleven. I know my rights; I'm not leaving until I get a cigarette!"

Another experimental patient, Aloysius, had been meek, cowardly. But after his dives, when another patient in the ward tried to bully him, Aloysius walked over and knocked his tormentor out of his wheelchair. The distressed nurses had to call the doctors, get X-rays taken, and write up detailed reports. Aloysius was a terrible patient. Now of course, Jacobs explains, the nurses recognized the value and importance of the senility therapy.

Despite a good preliminary showing plus additional positive reactions later, the senility study was small potatoes, a dinky experiment in the Veteran Administration's overall research program. It was a non-funded project, actually a parasite on the open-heart experiments which financed the hyperbaric chambers operation.

After ten months of experimenting with seniles, Jacobs was pulled up short. The hospital administration told her the old age study had cut into the hospital's research appropriation, and she had to stop immediately. Her experiments, they said, had taken from their money a total of $686!

Until she got her own research grant, she was not to run any more subjects. How does one get funded? She knew that meant getting published. She had planned to collect about thirty-five case histories before reporting on the experiment but had run only thirteen patients. So, she analyzed the data, wrote up the thirteen cases, and got published.

Her report, co-authored by Alvis, Winters and Small, appeared in the October 2nd, 1969, New England Journal of Medicine, and created a sensation in the hyperbaric field. This was the first systematic attempt to influence symptoms of senility by methods capable of producing marked improvement of cerebral oxygenation.

And how the Buffalo experiment succeeded! The eight patients who had breathed pure oxygen showed Improvement ranging from 35% to 300 percent. On the Wechsler Memory test their mean score rose from 76 to 103, their Bender-Gestalt from 10 to 41, and the Tien's 25 to 49.

There was no such improvement in the five controls. Their Wechsler actually dropped from 80.3 to 78.0, and the Tien's was unchanged at 90. Only their Bender-Gestalt average went up, from 6 to 15. The five control patients were subsequently given a full series on pure oxygen in the chamber, and also showed the same dramatic Improvement.

The clinical evidence was just as rewarding. The thirteen old men became more active, slept better, asked for magazines and newspapers to read, and, most importantly, resumed old habits of caring for themselves. Several were able to go home on visits, also a heartening development in later Buffalo experiments.

The Jacobs group realized their findings had barely scratched the surface of the possible role of hyperoxygenation in treating senility. The blood gas analyses showed big increases in arterial oxygen tensions in the treated patients, but the levels dropped back to normal within a half hour after the chamber sessions. Yet their Improvement in cognitive function persisted for several days, and in some cases for weeks.

And about the time the experiment was being reported in the New England Journal of Medicine, Jacobs presented the results to the American Psychological Association in Washington, DC and Winter carried the word to the Fourth International Congress on Hyperbaric Medicine in Sapporo, Japan.

Both reported marked clinical and psychological gains in their subjects but stressed there was no evidence that this improvement would persist, or that all senile people will benefit from hyperoxygenation even temporarily.

However, researchers across the country saw this as a highly promising avenue to follow in the urgent search for some means of relieving the mental miseries that haunt old age. Similar studies were promptly begun at Duke University Medical Center, New York University Medical Center, Mount Sinai Hospital in New York, Miami Heart Institute, Saint Luke's Hospital in Milwaukee and the Naval Hospital in Long Beach, California.

Jacobs was given a grant from the National Institute of Child Health and Human Development to resume her experiments, and by mid-1972 had tested approximately 100 subjects, with continued excellent results.

Although the medical literature has not previously contained anything as specific and precise in this field as the Buffalo experiment, two other researchers who preceded Jacobs had reached the same conclusion or had come close to it.

Dr Ross A. McFarland, the distinguished clinical psychologist and professor of aerospace health and safety at Harvard School of Public Health, began in the 1930s to investigate the role of oxygen want in the process of aging.

On an expedition into the Andes in Chile in 1935 to check the effects of high altitude living, McFarland discovered that "the most striking changes which occur in normal subjects at high altitude are precisely the ones that occur in persons as they grow older."

In the laboratory McFarland also observed that sensory and mental impairment which occurs in both normal and clinical subjects under oxygen deprivation simulate very precisely the behavioral changes observed in the aging process.

McFarland established that the well-known degeneration of many of the brain's higher functions—such as immediate recall, span of concentration, and insight—is accompanied by if not caused by impairment of cerebral vascular function. So are fainting, convulsions, and the senile or presenile degeneration of older persons.

He made similar observations in patients whose arterial oxygen saturation falls below certain levels whether the illness be heart failure, pneumonia, or any toxic agent influencing the red cells.

Even young people with severe anemia, McFarland discovered, show advanced symptoms of aging and senility. Likewise, he found close association between physiological reactions which are common to old age and hypoxia, or oxygen shortage. He identified those as the slowing of the basic resting frequency of EEG (shown on the brainwave recordings), impaired sensory functions such as adapting eyes to the dark, loss of ability to hear signs of high frequency, and increased reflex time.

McFarland raises an interesting possibility—that hypoxia may be the result rather than the cause of aging.

The other prior indication that HBO could have a beneficial effect on mental degeneration brought on by oxygen want emerged from Edgar End's years of clinical experience in the ancient little tank at Milwaukee County emergency hospital.

During the 1960s End had begun treating stroke victims in his tank, and dramatically helped them. He also had the distinct clinical impression that his stroke patients, most of whom were elderly, regained memory, and became brighter and happier.

In his ill-fated article on stroke, which was rejected in 1967 as "too absurd" for publication in The Journal of the American Medical Association, End wrote:

"The effect of hyperbaric oxygen on the psyche of a stroke patient is often dramatic. One refined, 56-year-old woman resisted rehabilitation efforts, responded to most stimuli with animal-like howls and uncontrolled sobbing, and resisted attempts to improve her appearance. We began treating her eight weeks after her stroke. Following her third treatment she smiled and tried to speak, and her nurses reported that when they placed a mirror before her and gave her a hairbrush, she spent long periods brushing and arranging her hair with her unparalyzed hand. She has made steady progress since that time, has returned to her home, is able to walk without a cane, communicates verbally and a limited fashion, and is now immaculately groomed and has become one of our most charming patients."

Eleanor Jacobs makes a point of calling attention to the prior work by McFarland and End. There is no feuding over credit. End was in the audience and loudly applauding in March 1972 at the Miami Heart Institute when she was given the first annual William McKnight $1,000 award for hyperbaric research.

"They (Jacobs and Alvis) deserve all the credit," End told me. "They are great scientists and humanitarians. If they hadn't come along, nobody would know anything about hyperbaric oxygen treatment of senility."

How long does this Improvement last? That is one of the biggest questions confronting researchers, and most of them are coming up with different answers. That should not be surprising because there is a great variance in patient age and the degree of deterioration; and hardly any hyperbarists give dives at precisely the same pressure, duration, frequency, or course span.

At Buffalo the improvement lasted on the average two weeks. But at the Miami (Florida) Heart Institute, Dr. Edwin Boyle reports his patients' memories perk up and stay improved for about six weeks. His treatment is given at 3 ATA but for only 30 minutes. Another difference is that he uses a one-patient Vickers chamber, small enough that the arteriosclerotic is also pressurized by the 100% oxygen environment he breathes inside the tank.

The Vickers chamber also is used at California's Long Beach Naval Hospital, where George Hart finds the revitalization of the seniles he treated lasted three to six months after the first treatment period. A second fifteen-day treatment produced improvement that lasted nine months to a year.

Milwaukee's Kindwall has been treating oldsters in his Saint Luke's Hospital Twin Chambers—called Bonnie and Clyde—but he doesn't believe this application of HBO is going to empty out the nursing homes. He thinks the prime candidate for this treatment—if it proves out satisfactorily—could be "the vigorous executive in his early 60s, working 10 hours a day—and who wants to keep what he's got."

The senility treatment has been given a new twist somewhat along this line at New York University Medical Center. Doctor Theobald Reich, director of the NYU Hyperbaric Department, sees a big difference between a patient racking up an impressive score in a psychological test and his improved functioning in real life.

In Reich's view this calls for devising specific programs for each patient to shore up the capabilities he has left and to build back his deficits. But the most unique part of his approach is to provide the input of "build-up" information as well as testing while the patient is undergoing oxygenation.

This requires one of the two research psychologists Drs. Yehuda Ben-Yishay or Leonard Diller, to go into the chamber with the patient to see if active coaching will help overcome senility and memory loss.

At a conference in August 1972 with Dr. Howard A. Rusk, director of NYU's Institute of Rehabilitation Medicine, Diller explained the process to me. Also present were Reich and Myron Youdin, a research scientist who was seeking better diagnostic uses of the tank.

Dillard does an analysis of memory and cognitive defects on each patient and attempts to do systematic training of memory functions in that area. For example, there may be a loss of memory for faces, dates, names, and abstract ideas. The NYU experimenters pinpoint this and then generate stimuli to these areas and try to develop objective ways of measuring any change.

Diller used the example of a high-level person with good thinking ability, and a still intact good IQ, but one who had developed a memory loss or had become slow at "catching on to things."

One technique is to give him seven editorial pages from The New York Times and have him read them and volunteer all the ideas he had gleaned. His effort is scientifically scored; then he is taken into the chamber to breathe pure oxygen while the Times experiment is repeated, and another test is taken to determine what changes have taken place in his mental functioning.

The obvious question is: what has been found so far?

Diller gave the answer heard over and over again from HBO researchers: "Some patients improve a great deal, some patients improve moderately, some patients don't improve at all."

"Why is that?" I asked.

"I can't give a simple answer," said Diller.

Rusk spoke up. "If we could see on the inside of their brain, then swim through the arterials, we would have a much better idea."

Reich explained that the research team wants first to prove the validity of their approach before launching fundamental work. The rehabilitation of senile people is very important for many views: moral, ethical, economic. But oxygen research, he says, is too expensive to merely demonstrate a trivial effect. The NYU team wants to be sure it produces something with clinical merit, an effect that is worthy of pursuit.

The problem, as Reich sees it, is to translate something done organically to the brain into behavior and determine the link between. A tall order, he believes, that will tax many minds and require perhaps several years to achieve.

Reich and his research teammates were concentrating on a new laboratory device that could be a medical breakthrough to open new diagnostic vistas far beyond the hyperbaric field.

They were putting together a non-invasive machine that would develop a three-dimensional picture of blood flow in the brain—small area by small area, something never before achieved.

In Buffalo a fantastic investigation of trace elements in the blood and their effect of cognition was started by Eleanor Jacobs.

Two hyperbaric centers which attempted to duplicate the Buffalo experiment ran into bad luck.

Dr Larry W. Thompson, professor of medical psychology at Duke, treated 22 seniles and found that only two improved significantly. Some of the control subjects actually went into convulsions, a report which alarmed Eleanor Jacobs. Her protocol was ultra-safe, and she couldn't understand the seizures. Later she determined what had gone wrong at Duke. Instead of using face masks, Duke had used an oxygen helmet. The control patients breathed a mixture of 10% oxygen and 90% nitrogen, and the mixture had somehow "layered" robbing these patients of adequate oxygen, fortunately all were being closely monitored and were revived when they got in distress.

At Mount Sinai School of Medicine in New York, Dr Alvin I. Goldfarb, associate professor of clinical psychiatry, undertook to pressurize a group of elderly patients just as Eleanor Jacobs had done. Things didn't go at all well. Everyone he put into the chamber got terribly nervous, and some panicked.

For a time, their behavior mystified him. Then he figured out the obvious explanation. All of his experimental patients were Jewish; they had become terrified because their poorly functioning minds had acquainted being locked inside his hyperbaric chamber with the horror of the Nazi gas chambers. Goldfarb did not try to continue his project.

Considering that the wretched burden of senility currently rests on about ten million American families, it is surprising that greater effort has not been expended in trying to do something to alleviate the curse. But most families seem to accept the problem. There is a widespread feeling nothing can be done to get rid of this unwelcome guest.

The tragedy is that HBO's potential help is so little known to ordinary people in everyday life. This unfortunate situation is dramatically illustrated by the poignant experience of Constance Warshoff of Livingston, New Jersey, with her mother, Mrs. Thelma Segel of East Orange, New Jersey.

Theirs was a fairly typical upper middle class family, active, intelligent, substantial: Mrs. Warshoff busy in home, clubs, politics; her father a New York public relations executive; her mother, once cheerful, gracious, and vivacious, broadcasting in the days of big radio over New York's WHN as Marsha Galett, operatic singer.

Then with scant warning, Constance Warshoff and her father felt themselves slowly becoming trapped by the cruel and baffling ordeal that the stride of time can bring to any of us. Mrs. Segel, in her early seventies, was losing her grip.

Constance Warshoff felt her heart being twisted every day by the wretched and relentless decline in her mother's mentation. Two seconds after she spoke to her mother, Mrs. Segel couldn't remember the conversation. She didn't know her son's name, in fact, didn't know how many children she had. She couldn't cook. Constance Warshoff saw her pick up a dishrag to wash the dishes; when she came back to the kitchen ten minutes later her mother was just standing there still holding the cloth. The daughter wanted to cry; it was so pitiful.

Like thousands of other dutiful children and concerned relatives, Mrs. Warshoff did not know where to turn for help. This seemed just something you had to endure.

Fate, luck, mere happenstance—whatever you choose to call it—happily intervened. In a doctor's office Mrs. Siegel's husband picked up a magazine and read a report on the Buffalo senility experiments. It seemed to offer hope and he asked his daughter to try to locate a hyperbaric center.

It is ironic that right in her hometown of Livingston the Saint Barnabas Medical Center operated one of the country's biggest HBO programs. But Mrs. Warshoff wasn't aware of it.

After checking around, Mrs. Warshoff found out about Saint Barnabas, and they took her mother there in January 1972. Mrs. Segel sat in the admitting office, her face swollen, her eyes dead-looking, not knowing or caring where she was, her daughter says.

During her first few days in the hospital, Mrs. Segal was very nervous and thought she was stranded, without money, in a hotel where she knew no one. The hospital doctors started her on a course of treatment, two dives daily for ninety minutes each at 3 ATA, breathing 100% oxygen by a mask.

The treatments went on about ten days, which means about thirty hours of hyperoxygenation, before Mrs. Warshoff noticed any change in her mother. She was sitting in Mrs. Segal's hospital room while she ate her lunch, talking to her mother's roommate.

Suddenly Mrs. Segal joined the conversation, and Mrs. Warshoff was so startled she went into a kind of state of shock and stopped talking. Mrs. Warshoff recalls:

"Mother said, 'Why did you stop talking; are you upset?' I said 'No', and she continued the conversation in a coherent manner I hadn't heard for two years. I just couldn't believe it."

I met Mrs. Warshoff while observing operations of the Saint Barnabas Chambers. Through a porthole she pointed out her mother who was taking a morning dive with other patients and told her story.

When Mrs. Segal came out of the tank, I spoke to her, and she responded pleasantly. Her eyes were bright, and she seemed in excellent condition. A nurse took her away in a wheelchair.

What even the belated discovery of HBO meant to just one family is succinctly reflected in a brief excerpt from my tape recorded interview with Mrs. Warshoff at the hospital:

Q. What do you think her condition is now?

A. Now she's a person again, she's not just a vegetable. She may not be able to function overly at home. But she won't be just sitting there.

Q. Why don't you think your mother's doctor knew about this and was able to propose it?

A. My mother's doctor said to forget it.

Q. He did?

A. I hate to tell you that.

Q. Why do you think he takes that attitude?

A. I don't know, but I don't think many doctors are oriented to it. They don't seem to care that they don't know.

Q. Do you think it was worth the expense?

A. I think it's worth everything; of course, in her case it is covered by Medicaid because she is over 65.

Q. Did your doctor tell you that it's a transitory effect, that what she gets here may not persist?

A. I couldn't care. What this has done for us as far as morale, and what it has done for her as a person, is worth even ten days of her life.

Six months later I telephoned Mrs. Warshoff to ask about her mother's condition. The daughter was very happy. Her mother was doing "nicely" by going to the hospital as an outpatient for one dive every Tuesday afternoon. Mrs. Warshoff said she looked better and took care of herself and stayed alone during the day except for a woman who came in about two hours.

Did she still feel the hyperbaric treatment had been beneficial and helpful?

"Oh, absolutely," said Mrs. Warshoff. "In every way. In every way."

12

SIDE EFFECTS–SEX AND I.Q.

Can the hyperbaric chamber do something for the libido? Increase sex drive in men past their prime? Give women firmer breasts... skin with fewer wrinkles or sags... longer fingernails?

Does it make an above normal IQ jump even higher? Turn graying hair dark again? Cause liver spots on the skin of oldsters to fade, or totally disappear? Sharpen up deteriorating eyesight?

These are questions that many hyperbaric doctors do not want to talk about although they are pretty sure the answers are affirmative. Their reticence stems from two primary concerns: first, fear that verbalizing such sensational findings prior to the firmest kind of scientific proof might expose them to ridicule in the medical profession; and second, that the uncertain course of HBO toward becoming an important tool of healing might be wrecked if the fickle public succumbed to unwarranted enticement of Fountain of Youth hoopla.

Because so much is unknown in the whole physiologic field, hyperbarists haven't been too surprised by the exotic side effects. The manifestations have surfaced more or less by accident. Certainly, in the beginning there was no organized attempt to demonstrate such a range of youthifying phenomena.

But in day-by-day clinical work, hyperbarists began independently stumbling onto unexpected and unexplained changes in their patient's sex life, looks, or brain power.

These developments so strained credulity that most doctors for a considerable time kept their findings quiet or ventured guarded disclosure only to close colleagues. And even as late as autumn 1972, reports on this aspect of HBO had not found their way into the medical literature; though it was clear that some reports eventually would be published.

Gradually the mood of reticence and caution broke down; doctors like to exchange juicy tidbits as much as the rest of us. Some of the dramatic incidents were too choice and startling to stay bottled up, and slowly leaked beyond private walls at several medical centers.

Finally, most of the findings reached an open discussion stage by physicians and professional conferences. These side effects were taken seriously and considered important facts —but this kind of discussion usually inspired the audience to a friendly but nervous titter.

Only a dozen physicians talked to me about the apparent upsurge and sexual drive as an aftermath of hyperbaric treatments. Half insisted on an off-the-record discussion, not wanting their names linked to the topic. They felt not enough is known yet about this particular aspect.

Sentiment was both strong and widespread for keeping all this hush-hush. One leading expert, Harry Alvis, editor of The Hyperbaric Medicine Newsletter, feels strongly that premature disclosure may mislead the public and also do harm to orderly development of the therapy. The September 1971 issue of the newsletter referred to certain unidentified experiments into these sexual aspects, and Alvis wrote that he joined others in suppressing such information until some means of confirming it on a truly scientific basis can be devised. He cautioned that some of this would be "tremendous grist for the mills of quackery to obtain."

Obviously, Alvis had in mind the public's gullibility for the fraudulent rejuvenating nostrums that rocketed into medical scandals—Dr Brinkley's goat gland operations, the patent medicine tonics for women, the alcoholic cures, cancer vaccines, the vitamin craze, etc., some of which still disturb organized medicine today.

Yet other equally prominent hyperbaric experts subscribe as much to candor as to caution. One of the most straightforward and outspoken is Hart of Long Beach Naval Hospital. A short time after he got into the field Hart began picking up hints of exotic side effects. When they emerged repeatedly and clearly, he talked as frankly about them as he did in reporting the success of his tanks in treating burns, stroke, or osteomyelitis.

Hart brought up the subject in his lecture under the aegis of the American distributor for the Vickers one-patient chambers, the Bethlehem Corp. of Bethlehem, Pennsylvania. He volunteered to tell the fascinating story connected with treatment of a patient who suffered osteomyelitis of the mandible (jawbone). The man was more than sixty years old. About four weeks after the patient began taking regular dives, his wife came to Hart and asked him to put her in the chamber, too.

"What for" the doctor asked.

"Well, I can't keep up with my husband's wifely demands."

The woman was explicit. It previously had been rare for them to have sex twice a year, and now her husband wanted intercourse about twice a week.

Hart said this patient also went around the wards at Long Beach Naval Hospital telling others about his rejuvenation. One who heard his testimony and got ideas from it was a patient seventy-two-years-old, who was recuperating from an operation for hemorrhoids. He falsified his own records, Hart said, got necessary tests and wrote his own orders for hyperbaric treatment, mimicking Hart's signature. He was given five dives before his ruse was found out.

That episode may seem redolent of the old Sunday supplement pseudo-science features, but Hart's observations cannot be lightly dismissed. Too many other doctors have discovered their older male hyperbaric patients also experienced a reawakened sex interest. This makes physiological sense, of course, to scientists who are studying the theory that aging results from a reduction of the endocrine function. The senility studies have already given clues that when HBO revitalizes the memory and general spirit of older people, men's sensual dreams likewise are rekindled.

Hart's clinical impressions are echoed by two of the most prominent senility researchers Edgar End of Milwaukee and Eleanor Jacobs of Buffalo, New York.

While interviewing Jacobs, I mentioned the incidents Hart described in his lecture and asked if any such side effects showed up on her treatment of old men, or of any wives complained.

Initially she was not aware of any such reaction for two good reasons; she had not inquired about it, and her beginning subjects chiefly were long-term patients who never left the hospital and had no wives.

The Buffalo Veterans Hospital nurses were the ones who complained about it—that the "boys" who had been given HBO treatments were pinching them, and ogling them, and trying to proposition them. Some of these boys were eighty!

Another staffer at the hospital explained that one of their hyperbaric patients, a retired Army colonel in his seventies, frankly told the physicians that his sexual prowess had been suddenly restored.

They believed him when a few weeks later he married again, picking a much younger woman, a woman in her thirties.

Over a period spanning three decades End has been probably the steadiest "customer" of his own hyperbaric chamber at Milwaukee's County Emergency Hospital, in the process of accompanying patients on dives, and in doing research projects under pressure.

From time to time End commented to colleagues in the field that the hyperoxygenation had increased his libido. This was passed on to me at a couple of hyperbaric centers, and I later put the question to him.

"Well," End said, "ordinarily I wouldn't mention that to anybody, but now that you have broken the ice—yes. I am as virile as I was at twenty-five."

Born in 1910, End is in his early sixties, the father of one son and seven daughters.

End's only evidence is empirical —just his clinical observations—but it is supported by similar manifestations in other patients. And End believes he has a valid method by which to measure his own stepped-up vitality. He uses as a comparison his own brother, seven years younger, and also a doctor. There is a marked difference between them. End says his brother is less vigorous and that is hair is thin while End's is thick and dark.

End has great confidence that HBO could be turned into a tremendously important "executive brush-up tool." He would like to see this technique applied at the top level of society, to individuals in positions of responsibility. He mentions diplomats, scientists, government officials, business leaders.

Big business is missing a good bet in HBO, End thinks. Top corporations insist on their key executives taking annual physical checkups at places like the Mayo Clinic. He wonders why they are not paying as much attention to preserving what these executives were really hired for—their mental skill.

HBO gave End another unusual dividend. For years he suffered from a crippling muscular impairment in one hand that prevented him from playing the violin. His fingers would not touch his palm. That condition changed and he attributed it to hyperoxygenation. Now he again plays the violin.

At Hennepin County General Hospital in Minneapolis, one HBO patient, about 68 years old, told the doctor that his sex life was rejuvenated. He was getting tank treatments for peripheral vascular lesions.

Hitchcock mentioned a case when I questioned him about libido increase. Hitchcock said there may be something to it, although this was the only instance in his experience, and it was without documentable evidence.

Nothing like that was experienced by any medical personnel working in the tank.

"But this one patient," said Hitchcock," he swore by it—really swore by it."

Skeptics want solid proof of what one disdainfully term "this horrendous stuff about sex". The confirmation may be on its way. For at one hyperbaric center, I discovered an extensive animal research project that is attempting to demonstrate the startling effect in a measurable way.

The investigation was at that time confidential, but the research team said they were getting the same indications George Hart had reported.

When hyperbaric patients at this hospital first began happily announcing their restored sex drive, the researchers were not impressed.

For months they ignored the talk, knowing that a lot of sexual feelings are psychological. How could they be sure the patients didn't just have a better sense of physiologic well-being? They obviously would feel more like exerting themselves, but the medical staff couldn't tell what was real and what was brag. As one researcher smirked: "There's a big difference between getting an erection and maintaining an erection."

But the staff finally decided to undertake animal studies. The first experiment was with rats. Old rats, of course. Could HBO light the fires again in elderly, deteriorated, retired male breeding rats? In the rat world sex is usually a nocturnal activity, so in a darkened cage the researchers placed one of their old rats and separated him by only a clear plexiglass partition from a healthy young female rat. The old rat could look but not touch.

There were a battery of these blacked-out cages. At intervals, a dim red light was turned on and the plexiglass barrier was removed. The researchers played Peeping Tom and did a frequency count on attempts at copulation.

There weren't many. So, the old rats were given a series of hyperbaric treatments. Then another dim red light trysting opportunity. This time the old rats became amorous, and the frequency count was startlingly high. But the researchers were dissatisfied; they doubted their statistics. It was difficult with rats to tell what actually a real consummation was and what was merely an attempt at copulation.

One member of the research team suggested using rabbits. "With rabbits," he said, "when the male actually has an orgasm, he slaps his feet on the floor and generally falls backward. There's no question what's for real and what's not.

They acquired a number of very old, retired breeding type male rabbits that were beyond their life expectancy and started over again.

The beat-up looking, doddering male rabbits were divided into Groups A and B. Each old rabbit was placed in a cage separated by a plexiglass barrier from a healthy young bunny. Twice a day the barriers went up so the researchers could see if the oldsters attempted copulation.

It was, in the words of one researcher, "Dullsville". The old rabbits showed no interest in the young females.

So, Group A was given hyperbaric treatment, pressurized in 100% oxygen. Group B was the control. It got the same pressurization but in an atmosphere containing just 10% oxygen, which in the tank was the equivalent of only normal room air. Thus, Group B actually got no HBO.

Again, each old rabbit was given the same twice-a-day opportunity to copulate. The researchers kept score. Group A was indeed sexier; and Group B was not.

Group A's copulation was up, up, up, up! Statistically up, said the chief researcher. This was considered a small, inconclusive sample and the project was being broadened to seek more convincing data. But as one member of the team pointed out, there already was some rather convincing proof — "a lot of baby bunnies down there in our cages that were just not supposed to be."

How can needed scientific proof be obtained in human studies? Not likely by assigning research associates to spy on a patient's sex life. The current emphasis is on the practical side, measuring sex hormone excretion. This is a reasonably uncomplicated procedure and is recognized as valid by medical scientists.

There seems little doubt that HBO does restore sexual potential. Testosterone levels were found markedly higher among old men receiving hyperbaric treatment in senility studies. And George Hart also discovered a similar influence on the sexual nature of women. In his Bethlehem Corp. lecture, Hart remarked that he had no problem getting human volunteers. He added: "And I might say from my wife's aspect and from my own aspect, plus my three secretaries who volunteered, the head of ENT, the head of oral surgery and their wives, we found that this does accentuate estrogen and androgen output. That definitely happened; it makes an improvement."

Eyes are very sensitive to high concentrations of oxygen. HBO seems to improve the vision of elderly patients, although it can be dangerous to put babies in the tank. Premature infants may develop a condition known as retrolental fibroplasia, which is formation of opaque tissue behind the lens that can cause detachment of the retina and arrest of eye growth.

Reports of eyesight Improvement among adults are commonplace. On this subject End observed that some patients voluntarily report better vision. His most dramatic results were in a registered nurse who had retinal histoplasmosis (infection of the retina) with such reduction in vision that she could not read the route sign on the front of the bus when standing on the sidewalk in front of it. By the time she finished treatment she could identify her children a block away. She returned to work full time in the hospital.

On the other hand, at the Norwalk, Connecticut, Symposium, Hart cautioned that people who are myopic (nearsighted), would find their vision deteriorating following repetitive hyperoxygenation. His hospital's ophthalmologist made a study of tank patients and found eighty who had changes in their refraction.

New York University's Reich says his eyesight has gotten worse since he has been working in the chamber; but he shies away from this sort of observation. He feels this should be gone into in some sort of scientific way.

In his stroke and senility paper that was "too absurd" to print in the Journal of the American Medical Association, End described the case of a 66-year-old physician who had suffered a stroke with severe hemiplegia (paralysis of one side of the body), fifty-one days before beginning hyperbaric treatment. End wrote:

After his third treatment he was able to overcome marked toe-drop and raise his hands above his head. After his sixth treatment he was elated by the growth of strong dark hair into the margins of his bald spot. The cause of this regrowth is not clear. It probably represents an endocrine effect of the hyperbaric oxygen. It also resulted in a large number of previously reluctant and alopecic physicians suddenly volunteering to serve as controls by inhaling oxygen under pressure with their patients.

The hair darkening phenomenon was neither wanted nor appreciated by one hyperbaric patient. Hart's research nurse, Alice Gaul, recounted the case of an elderly woman with strikingly beautiful silver hair treated at Long Beach Naval Hospital. When black threads began streaking her shiny coiffure, she was furious!

Hart had made the comment that HBO appears to firm women's breasts. I brought this up to the women on his research staff.

"Yes, it does," one said. The other nodded in agreement.

"Can you testify to it yourselves?" I inquired, knowing both had taken a number of dives in various experimental studies.

They gave no answer.

Later Mrs. Gaul commented that the treatment generally has a lot of Fountain of Youth side effects. Older people, she said, experience a tightening of the skin. I asked why.

"Just more resiliency, I suppose," she said, "It seems to happen all over the body."

Several medical centers are attempting careful analysis of just how much an already superior intelligence can be bolstered. Hart has used himself and his wife as guinea pigs in such experimentation. Before starting on a series of dives his IQ was measured at 132. After 15 treatments in a single-blind exploratory study his IQ went up to at least 143.

Dr. Allen Edwards of the Veterans Administration Center in Los Angeles administered the IQ tests—the Wechsler Adult Intelligence Scale, known in psychologist's surface as the WAIS test.

The reason Hart didn't know precisely how much his brain power increased is that the top score possible was 143.

Hart's IQ remained at 143 for nine months. At that point a test showed he had fallen back to his previous level of 132. He promptly undertook a new series of dives and once again his IQ went up.

Long before he became a physician, Milwaukee's Eric Kindwall experimented as a youngster with a hyperbaric tank's effect on mentation. His boyhood fondness for scuba diving, a sport that requires a broad understanding of the oxygen and pressure principles, lead Kindwall into a protégé relationship with End.

Kindwall began scuba diving with very meager gear—a war-surplus gas mask and a bicycle pump. But he read a lot of books on the subject. In 1956 he got interested in the physiological aspects and suggested to Dr. End that he would like to measure IQ change at a pressure of a hundred feet. He wanted to see what nitrogen narcosis did.

Kindwall used the Otis test and the Minnesota Multiphasic Personality Inventory. He spent most of the summer getting the chamber ready and had time to only run six men before the summer ended. The data was never published, but Kindwall says it was interesting, explaining:

In terms of raw point scores, the most intelligent men went down the most, and the least intelligent men, who had the least to lose, went down the least. We never knew what that meant, if anything.

The use of hyperbaria as a preventive device toward off normal mental slowdown is under study at Miami Heart Institute. Their primary program is aimed at reversing deterioration in seniles, but these researchers are also trying to gauge the desirability of brush-up therapy for executives in their 40s or 50s.

"Or perhaps younger," says Dr. Edwin Boyle, the Institute's research director.

Boyle says it has repeatedly been proven that the human mental ability peaks at age 25 and starts downhill, and thus a 45-year-old man has already 20 years down the slope. Boyle believes middle-aged people learn to compensate in a variety of ways— "such as getting a better secretary," he says, seriously—and often show no apparent loss of mental ability.

If HBO does turn out to be a panacea for old age's mental impairment, the Miami researchers foresee drastic changes in society as it exists today.

Throughout world history, Boyle observes, the elderly have been the leaders—the seers, the visionaries, the highly respected. Nowadays, he says, whether they want to go or not, they are usually kicked out at age sixty-five.

Up to now the mental decline that comes with advancing age has been considered irreversible, Boyle says; adding the good news that this does not have to be so in a high percentage of instances. He urges researchers to get busy and find out more about the problem.

The mystery of unknown side effects is of great interest to the hyperbaric team at New York University. Reich ponders the possible chronic effects on patients given prolonged treatment; there are so many unknowns in this area experimenters should proceed with caution.

Does the idea of the executive brush-off strike them as having merit?

The psychologist, Diller, thinks it's possible, with a little imagination. It would be very exciting to see old people take a whiff of something and give an elixir effect to minds that are beginning to slip. But he also fears a possible backlash that might sour the public on the field of unwise experiments prove fruitless.

The best way to find the answers, in Reich's opinion, is to pursue a careful one and one situation—one patient, one investigator. Otherwise, there is always danger of wild-eyed speculation.

Is there any feeling in the NYU program that organized medicine is too conservative in accepting the clinical benefits of hyperbaric therapy?

Reich pointed out that this involves the "other part" of human nature, and the doctor's nature. They're only human, he observes, and so everyone concerned must strike a happy balance.

"In medicine," he says, "you should be conservative in publishing success; you should be imaginative in pursuing work."

13

POISON...FIRE...AND EXPLOSION!

It would be foolhardy to try to deny or even soft-pedal the very obvious and serious hazards associated with the use of oxygen under high pressure. As in other effective therapeutic procedures, inherent dangers lurk in both the necessary medical machinery and also within the drug itself.

No one needs to be told that any pressure vessel—an auto tire, a kitchen pressure cooker, or a sturdy hyperbaric tank—can be pushed too far and forced to explode.

Or that any oxygen-rich atmosphere greatly intensifies the risk of destructive fire.

Less well understood are hyperoxygenation's physiological side effects, which can be startling. The truth is that life giving oxygen can turn rapidly into a deadly poison!

If a man breathes oxygen under too high pressure too long his central nervous system will become impaired and throw him into convulsions. His lungs will also suffer, becoming toxic and tending to thicken into liver-like globs, and fail.

Human physiology is so delicate that a powerful stimulus like oxygen can derange its delicate balance and make the body go haywire and try to destroy itself for unknown reasons.

Toxicity is the chief worry, because doctors haven't determined fully its cause and effect. Debate flared over adverse theories, such as whether HBO might activate dormant cancer cells and cause metastases to spread. Some radiologists thought they saw this in their patients, but other specialists contend strongly that no firm evidence supports such fears.

Everyone is in agreement oxygen use requires utmost caution; and events of the past decade illustrate the point.

Since 1962 a scattering of unfortunate accidents in hyperbaric chambers in clinical use have killed half a dozen patients or doctors. And in the broader and more hazardous experimental area of space and undersea exploration, the death toll is woefully much higher. One horrifying mishap literally stunned the entire scientific world—the January 1967 fire in the oxygen-filled Apollo Command Module that snuffed out the lives of three US astronauts.

Despite this dark side, hyperbaric oxygenation—applied by a competent physician and within known limits—is nonetheless considered safe, probably no riskier than getting an X-ray or letting some nurse give you a penicillin shot.

Present-day tanks are built to meet rigid design and structural standards, with safeguards against accidental overpressurization. Obviously, no hospital is looking for a holocaust, so chamber fire hazards today are virtually nonexistent.

And fortunately, the hyperbaric physician can easily circumvent the dangerous physiological side effects merely by limiting the oxygen pressure and duration of exposure—two readily controllable variables in the treatment.

What are the safe limits? Kindwall of Milwaukee limits exposure of a patient breathing 100% oxygen to approximately two hours at 2 ATA or 90 minutes at 3 ATA. Hyperbarists and other hospitals generally observe about the same limits, halting the dive at that point to let the patient "rest" and breathe normal air.

When these exposures are alternated with periods of air breathing, explains Kindwall, the patient can be treated repetitively for hours or days with safety. Observing these precautions, pulmonary oxygen toxicity and central nervous system symptoms are a rarity, he says. And most experts concur.

There is seldom any reason to risk dangerous extremes in clinical hyperbaria. Researchers long ago clearly established the danger zones and every physician in the field makes certain that he holds his patient well short of excessive oxygenation.

Yet for all the diligent investigation, more remains unknown about oxygenation then is known. Its secrets, if found out, might go a long way toward unraveling the greater mystery of precisely why our marvelous bodies can behave in such abnormal fashion.

Medical ignorance in the area of oxygen toxicity is astounding, considering that the danger was first recognized by Priestley and Lavoisier two hundred years ago. Experiments have been steadily undertaken with hundreds of thousands of laboratory animals—rats, rabbits, birds, calves, pigs, dogs—and the actual mechanism of either of the two toxic manifestations still eludes explicit explanation.

One problem in getting answers is that man never reacts totally in the same manner as any experimental animal. Thus, the facts established in the research lab may not stand up in treating humans.

Further, one man may not respond to oxygenation precisely as does his brother. And more disturbing, according to Dr. John W. Bean, the University of Michigan physiologist, one individual may show a wide variation from day to day or even hour to hour in his own tolerance to oxygen.

With his microscope, Bean studied anatomical changes in the pulmonary mechanism after oxygen overdose. He came to the conclusion that the cause of toxicity was a complicated, inconstant involvement of a combination of factors. When pressurized oxygen enters the lungs it produces changes in the membrane and blood vessels, capillaries, surfactant (internal moisture ratio), carbon dioxide accumulation, enzymes, neurogenic factors (the telegraph lines to the brain), the hormones, and many more parts of the anatomy.

Simplifying his medical jargon, you might compare development of oxygen toxicity to an amateur trying to open a bank vault. He spins the knobs on the lock, sending pins and tumblers inside the door gyrating every which way. Not just one piece, but several, must drop precisely into place and in sequence—as per the combination—before the door will swing open.

In much the same way, the precise "combination" that regulates the proper function of your lungs can be thrown easily out of kilter. One pulmonary mechanism is incredibly complex! It also is so delicately balanced that a slight decrease in the oxygen content of the air we breathe will trigger a respiratory control alert.

Curiously, such trouble can start from false as well as true danger signals—when the brain gets mixed up about whether we are getting too little or too much oxygen!

A sudden decrease in the air's oxygen content, for example, immediately flashes a warning to our internal sensors that control respiration. The working of these wonderful physiological sentries is not fully understood by medical scientists, but they are known to be alert and edgy, ever on guard to help the body defend itself. It takes very little to make them hit the panic button.

To compensate for too little oxygen, these respiratory regulators start a whole array of adjustments—in the lungs, in the central nervous system, and especially in the body's vast network of blood vessels. Fearing the body is about to be starved for oxygen, the sensors direct the heart to speed up and pump faster so a greater blood flow will carry what oxygen is available more quickly to the cells.

In the reverse situation, when a person inhales air with a high oxygen content—as in an HBO chamber—the respiratory sensors interpret this, too, as a possible threat that might produce oxygen toxicity. So, the brain messages the heart to slow down, so as to pump less blood and avoid drenching the cells with an oxygen overdose. Also, this alert causes the blood vessels to constrict, further slowing circulation.

Such a false signal is likely, of course, when any patient is put in an HBO chamber. In a case of gas gangrene, for instance, the deceased cells would desperately need the hyperoxygenation, yet the respiratory sensors would not comprehend that fact. To counteract this problem, hyperbaric physicians frequently administer vasodilators—drugs that enlarge the arteries in veins—prior to a patient's dive.

The false signal can be fatal quickly to laboratory animals. When exposed to abnormal oxygen concentrations, such guinea pigs usually develop what physicians term hyperoxic anoxia, which means paradoxically, absence of oxygen in body tissues despite an excess of oxygen entering the lungs.

Once our respiratory machinery is thrown out of kilter by any alert, the disorder is extremely difficult to bring under control. The slowdown of the heart and constriction of arteries and veins bring on a general sludging of blood. The slower circulation does not properly carry off carbon dioxide and metabolites (garbage released by the cells in the metabolism process).

Normally, carbon dioxide in the blood is at a harmless low concentration. But the sludging starts a dangerous carbon dioxide build-up. This congratulate rise to a level that produces a frightening dual effect, both excitation and depression. One hazard of this dual effect is that the patient may actually lose his instinct to breathe; this is called apnea—transient cessation of the breathing impulse.

The opposite result is that the carbon dioxide build-up stimulates deeper respiration which in turn greatly increases the concentration of carbon dioxide in the sludged blood, worsening a poisonous condition that can induce convulsions and even death.

Not only does such sensor confusion vainly overtax the body system of immediate defenses, the long-range hormone protective balance can also be wrecked. If the so-called hypophyseal-adrenal cortical axis picks up a false danger signal, it pours stimulating agents out of the pituitary and adrenal glands in great volume. This releases a flood of cortisone which, when not actually required, and quickly used up, inflicts long-term damage throughout your body.

Once the patient stumbles into this toxicity trap, both he and his doctor become increasingly helpless. Nothing is any longer normal. The body is confused, actually attacking instead of defending itself. The physician cannot rely on administration of standard drugs and medication to produce customary effects. Even giving a patient anesthesia inside a pressure chamber can cause unpredictable exotic effects that might intensify his toxicity.

If all those problems aren't scary enough, there is also the mysterious off effect. Doctors use this term to describe what happens to a patient who tolerates steady hyperbaric pressure with no trouble—until decompression starts. Then he suffers severe convulsions (not believed associated with the bends).

Curiously oxygen toxicity does not seem to adversely affect the heart. And if harmful pressure is arrested without undue delay, recovery usually is rapid. Dr. A. R. Behnke, Jr., of San Francisco, the great Navy experimenter, noted this in reporting on a dog he subjected to 6 ATA and forced into 34 separate convulsions over a sixty-day span. Brought out into the air, the dog would stagger about blindly but recover fully in ten to twenty minutes.

"There is no pharmacologic or other agent," marveled Behnke, "that can so drastically disrupt body economy (meaning its system of operation), and yet be followed by apparently complete recovery."

Despite available safeguards, the hyperbaric therapists have encountered clinical disappointments. Patients have been lost, while the doctors found themselves confounded by the physiological quirks of high pressure oxygenation.

On August 25th, 1963, a 17 year-old-girl, desperately ill from a bungled abortion, was brought to Duke University Medical Center—to become "the first reported occurrence of irreversible oxygen toxicity in man."

The six physicians involved—Drs. Robert L. Funson, Herbert A. Saltzmann, Wirt W. Smith, Robert E. Whalen, Suydam Osterhout, and Roy T. Parker—reported the case in the August 19th, 1965, issue of The New England Journal of Medicine to alert other doctors to the fact that serious hazards of therapeutic hyperbaric oxygenation are not fully appreciated.

From the start, the girl looked like a goner. She already had been ill a week with overwhelming peritonitis and septicemia from her pelvic infection. Despite insertion of surgical drains, use of antibiotics, blood transfusion and three days of continuous hypothermia that cooled her body to 34 or 35 degrees C., the girl seemed to be dying.

As a last resort, the doctors decided to try using Duke's relatively brand new hyperbaric chamber. The girl, kept packed in ice, was moved into the tank. She was pressurized to 2 ATA, but events didn't go smoothly. She repeatedly choked on fluids, so a tracheostomy was performed to permit her to breathe through a tube inserted into her windpipe. She was kept under pressure about eight hours at 2 ATA, plus one hour at 3 ATA.

Next day she was pressurized on 100% oxygen for two hours at 3 ATA, and soon appeared stronger. On the third day the girl breathed pure oxygen for two hours at 2.5 ATA and that dive ended uneventfully. But half an hour later, back in her hospital bed, the girl suddenly had a convulsion, became confused, and partially paralyzed. Three minutes later she had a second seizure.

The doctors were not certain what to make of this unexpected development. It didn't look like a manifestation of oxygen toxicity, but rather as though a cerebral air embolism (bubble) in the blood was blocking circulation to the brain, or the central nervous system had suffered a "hit" from the bends.

Either disorder required immediate recompression—the long, drawn-out Class 4 US Navy procedure that meant pressurizing immediately to 6 ATA for one hour in chamber air, and then gradually stepping down the pressure back to sea level over the next 38 hours.

This was undertaken at once and in about two hours the patient's seizures had subsided and the paralysis disappeared. Three and a half hours later the doctors inside the tank fed pure oxygen into her endotracheal tube; and in fifteen minutes she again went into convulsion. They shut off the oxygen immediately and the seizure ended.

For the next thirteen and a half hours of routine decompression the girl remained comfortable, "and then acute respiratory distress suddenly developed, with manifestations of gross air hunger, fish-mouth breathing, restlessness and hypotension." This was the worst kind of new crisis. The doctors put her back on pure oxygen, and for the next ten hours anxiously administered medicine to both stimulate the adrenal glands and raise the blood pressure.

The decompression step-downs continued, but this situation was hopeless. "Twenty minutes after decompression to 1.3 ATA," said the doctors' report, and thirty-seven hours after the beginning of the prolonged decompression procedure, the patient died.

The autopsy cleared up part of the mystery. The lungs were congested and edematous, with a liver-like appearance; many lung secretions contained thickened hyaline membranes; no section had escaped severe involvement, and some areas had hemorrhaged. Cause of death clearly was pulmonary oxygen toxicity.

The Duke doctors wound up their case history with this admonition to other clinicians:

In view of the present limited knowledge, extreme care in the application of hyperbaric oxygenation should be observed. Until more information concerning the biochemistry, pathogenesis, pharmacology and prevention of oxygen toxicity is accumulated, exposures to hyperbaric oxygenation should be brief.

Virtually every other major oxygen-pressurized chamber tragedy in the last ten years has occurred in military or space agency test facilities—and involve fire or explosion, or both. In a strict sense they should not be considered black marks on the hyperbaric medical record, but nevertheless those calamities originated from the same kind of engineering hazards which must be guarded against in all pressure chambers.

NASA officials had a big red circle on their calendars around January 27th, 1967. It was to be another milestone in the race to the moon—the day for the first "plugs-out" test of the Apollo spaceship.

Into the cone-shaped command module that was the nose of the 218-foot rocket standing on Launching Pad 34 at Cape Kennedy climbed three astronauts. They locked the double hatches and settled back on cockpit couches in silvery space suits. The entire cabin was pressurized with pure oxygen.

At 2:50 pm Lieutenant Colonel Virgil (Gus) Grissom, 40, Lieutenant Colonel Edward White, 36, and Lieutenant Commander Roger Chaffey, 31, began a dress rehearsal for their scheduled February 21st blast-off. This run-through of their make-believe launch would keep them twisting dials and throwing switches until 8 PM. NASA technicians on the towering scaffold hovered alongside, monitoring the astronauts' simulation, communicating by radio.

Things went smoothly until, at 6:31 PM, a voice cried from inside the capsule: "Fire aboard the spacecraft!"

Two technicians saw a blinding flash through the cabin windows. Heavy smoke began seeping out. One technician raced to open the hatch. Scorching heat drove him back. Others snatched up asbestos gloves and masks and dared the heat. After a furious six-minute struggle, the hatch was sprung.

It was too late. Three charred bodies lay in the couches. The astronauts never really had any chance to escape.

This disaster stunned the public; and reminded hyperbarists of the ever-present danger they must guard against—use of oxygen in a sealed chamber.

What went wrong? Why did fire break out? Was there some mysterious new or unknown hazard?

Everybody wanted answers. Congress and the space agency investigated. Was the use of oxygen too dangerous? "For more than seven years," said Time, "during 1,024 hours of successful space flight and thousands of ground tests and pure oxygen atmospheres, NASA's reasoning seemed sound... But in 14 terrible seconds... NASA's carefully considered decision had been thrown open to question."

NASA was unable to pinpoint the exact cause of the fire. It probably was ignited by an electrical wire whose Teflon insulation may have worn thin from chafing by repeated opening and closing of an equipment compartment door. Grissom's wife and two sons blamed North American Rockwell Corp., and sued for $15,000,000 million dollars, contending the spacecraft was defective. The manufacturer settled these suits in March 1972 for $350,000.

Even so monumental a tragedy did not shake NASA's faith in the use of a properly safeguarded oxygen atmosphere. All subsequent space cabins—including the first moon lander on July 20th, 1967—were filled with oxygen.

Just four days after the Apollo fire, tragedy hit the space cabin simulator at Brooks Air Force Base, Texas, where 16 rabbits were undergoing a test to determine their tolerance to a 100% oxygen atmosphere at a simulated altitude of 15,000 feet.

Airman Second Class William F. Bartley, Jr., twenty, of Indianapolis, and Airman Third Class Richard G. Harmon, twenty-one, of Auburn, New York, had gone inside to draw blood samples. In a few minutes the technician on duty outside the tank heard a ruffling sound in his earphones. He sprang up, looked in a porthole, and saw flames. The noise was the airmen making a break for the door, which they couldn't open.

The technician immediately flooded the chamber with air, but it took four minutes to open the hatch and drag out the two airmen. Gravely burned, both died in a few hours.

Congressional investigators severely criticized Brook's safety precautions as grossly inadequate. The airmen had not been instructed how to use two fire extinguishers inside the tank, there were no extinguishers outside the tank, and no one kept watch on the men inside the chamber. Officials at Brooks, Congress was told, thought that the real danger to the blood samplers were such things as decompression sickness (the bends) rather than the risk of fire.

Stunned by back-to-back dual tragedies that had cost five lives, the Air Force Aerospace Medicine Division immediately suspended all experiments with pure oxygen pending full investigation.

The oxygen atmosphere was not at fault. The cause of the Texas fire was sheer negligence. A careful check of the work-lamp cords in the tank would have saved the two lives. One cord was worn and in touching the aluminum floor had caused an electric arc, investigators decided.

What made this carelessness seem even worse was that five years earlier there also had been a spark-caused fire during a pure oxygen experiment in the same chamber. Two Air Force captains managed to get out alive in that September 9th, 1962, blaze, suffering only smoke inhalation. But that incident's "warning" apparently was ignored.

Fire also had broken out November 17th, 1962, in the oxygen-filled pressure chamber at Philadelphia's Naval Air Material Center. Three Navy officers and a Marine flier were inside undergoing routine tests of high-altitude adaptability.

One, Lieutenant Commander Francis Highly of Charlotte, North Carolina, was a Navy physician. With him were Ensign Al Gershtenschlaiger of Wadsworth, Ohio, Ensign Stephen Marshall of Melrose, Massachusetts, and Marine First Lieutenant Gary Gebo of Stockton, California.

A spark set off the blaze—but luck was on their side. They managed to scramble out, escaping with only first and second degree burns on their arms and legs.

The Navy's worst pressurized oxygen fire broke out at 9:53 AM February 16th, 1965, in Experimental Diving Chamber No. 6 in the Washington, DC, Navy Yard—and immediately threw a scare into hospital administrators from coast to coast who were just then trying to decide whether to install hyperbaric chambers.

Boatswain Mate Second Class Frederick W. Jackson, thirty-seven, of Brandywine, Maryland, and Engineman First Class John P. Youmans, thirty-seven, of Corals Hills, Maryland, had just finished a two-hour test dive to a simulated depth of 250 feet, breathing 15% oxygen and 85% helium. They emerged from the "wet pot," and crawled through a tunnel into another tank to begin an eight-hour-and-forty-two-minute decompression.

Technicians outside increased the oxygen content to 3 percent. An electric "scrubber" was withdrawing carbon dioxide from the tank. The men stripped off diving suits and put on terry cloth robes. The next instant one cried into the intercom: "We got a fire in here!"

Those outside saw through the porthole a yellow-orange flame about four inches wide shooting two feet high out of the scrubber. In a moment a flash engulfed the tank and swirling smoke blotted out the tragic scene.

Despite impossible odds against rescue, two Navy divers, Boatswain Mate First Class James R. Taylor, thirty-four, of Forest Heights, Maryland, and Machinery Repairman First Class Richard Garrahan, twenty-nine, of Washington, crawled into the tunnel and tried to fight their way through 800-degree heat to their doomed buddies.

A ball of fire belched out the inner latch. Garrahan stumbled backward and fell into the "wet pot"—an accident that saved his life because he was able to breathe oxygen near the surface of the water. Taylor retreated safely.

It was a full hour before the bodies of Jackson and Youmans could be recovered.

This was another tragedy that need not have happened. The paper filter in the scrubber was at fault. It was found to contain a kerosene residue that could produce spontaneous combustion under the tank's heat conditions. But somebody had slipped up—the divers weren't warned about this hazard.

Once again, the hyperbaric doctors ground their teeth at the senseless carelessness that might cause the public to doubt the safety of oxygen therapy. Hospitals and manufacturers should reevaluate all their safety standards, suggested the authoritative Fire Journal. Because the facts were very plain—once a fire breaks out in a pressurized chamber there really isn't enough time to rescue anybody. The surest safeguard would be eagle-eyed vigilance against all hazards—and prevent fires from ever starting!

Within a two-year period two one-patient medical hyperbaric chambers exploded, and a third caught fire. The blaze occurred at a hospital in Gifu, Kyoto, Japan, on October 10th, 1967. A forty-year-old clerk had been put in the small tank after an ulcer operation for continued bleeding —which seems a peculiar reason.

A nurse noticed the fire through a porthole. But it took thirty minutes to lower the pressure and open the door. The clerk was dead. The fire's cause couldn't be determined.

Dr. Daniel A. Tobin had about as close a call as anyone would want. At the University Hospital in Madison, Wisconsin, he was investigating the effect of radiation on advanced cancer patients treated while in a hyperbaric chamber. He was using a two-by-seven foot chamber manufactured by the Bethlehem Corp. of Bethlehem, Pennsylvania. It was sheathed by a clear, supposedly shatterproof canopy (supplied by a plastics company) through which X-ray and cobalt could be administered.

On May 2nd, 1968, the sixth patient of the day—a sixty-year-old man with advanced bladder cancer—was placed in the chamber. The pressure was slowly raised to 3 ATA. Twenty-nine minutes later, while Tobin bent over the tank adjusting the X-ray Focus, the chamber blew apart.

Jagged chunks of plastic whistled to every corner of the room. Tobin was hurled eight feet into a steel bookcase and fell unconscious with a shattered jaw, facial cuts, and injuries to spine and shoulder. The nurse's forehead was gashed. The sudden decompression collapsed the patient's lungs and powdered him with plastic dust. The hospital's "Blue Cart" emergency team rushed in and relieved the patient's pneumothorax. Ten days later he was well enough to resume his radiation treatment.

But Tobin called it quits. He terminated the entire experimental study—incidentally finding no marked difference in radiation with or without HBO. He later became Associate Director, Radiation Center, University of Louisville (KY) School of Medicine.

Back about 1959, Coyoacan Hospital in Mexico City purchased a portable, lightweight, one-man collapsible chamber, initially designed as a diver decompression tank by Draeger in Germany. The hospital used it about five hundred times for hyperbaric treatment.

On February 13th, 1969, a very ill forty-five-year-old man with a severe brain injury was put in the chamber and quickly pressurized to 3 ATA, according to an account from Dr. Michael Crist of Mexico City published in The Hyperbaric Medicine Newsletter. About five minutes later the tank suddenly flew apart. The bottom half knocked a big hole in a brick wall and the top part shot forward and hit a physician and an orderly. Both were seriously hurt.

The patient was left lying on the table where the chamber had been resting—mercifully dead. Autopsy disclosed his spine was fractured, both arms shattered, sternum disarticulated from the ribcage, clavicles broken, intercostal muscles torn, and both legs ruptured. In contrast, the organs of the abdomen and pelvis were normal as were the lower limbs.

Six months later, the injured physician, Dr Gabriel Diaz de Urdanivia, died.

Seeking a probable cause investigation, investigators found part of an L-shaped rim on the chamber's head section had somehow unfolded and blamed the accident on metal fatigue.

Details are available on a dozen or so other accidents and pressure chambers, but they are primarily related to underwater experiments—such as the March 22nd, 1968, fire aboard the USS Chanticleer that killed a diver and a Navy officer, and the November 1971 deaths of four Russian oceanauts in a diving bell.

Diligent research covering the last decade discloses no additional "horror stories" involving strictly medical hyperbaric chambers, although some physicians say candidly there obviously have been many incidents of undetected oxygen toxicity from HBO therapy.

But if this chapter has severely jolted your faith in the practical safety of modern hyperbaric facilities, operated by competent physicians, pause a moment and consider the multitudinous hazards abounding in everyday life.

Or even more specifically meditate on medicines' over-all track record. Even the conscientious good doctors willing to break their backs trying can't win 'em all.

14

RESEARCH AND GOVERNMENT MONEY

The federal government now pays for nearly two-thirds of all medical research in the United States. Thus Washington, where the money is, largely determines the tempo and dimension of studies into the usefulness of hyperbaric chambers.

Scads of research money is available. Any promising project can get government financial support if it passes muster with scientific review boards, perhaps faster if the subject intrigues taxpayers enough to talk it up with their congressman.

Better health has become a national mania, and dollars have been shoveled into medical R & D at an ever-faster clip for the last quarter century. As recently as 1950 only $161 million dollars was spent from both public and private sources in this quest. The current yearly outlay is up to an estimated $3.3 billion, of which federal agencies administer about two billion.

Even that is not the full financial picture. This research cost does not take into account an additional $3 billion a year spent on medical facilities construction, an item which also has a distinct bearing on the availability and use of HBO.

Though footing most of the bills, Uncle Sam tries to keep his guiding hand very light on medical research ventures. In general, biomedical investigators sponsored by the government are on their own, experimenting in their laboratories and clinics across the land. This easy partnership is meant to guarantee competent researchers free rein for their intellectual curiosity and Inspirations without red tape or bureaucratic interference.

The fountainhead of most medical research spending is the National Institutes of Health, an agency so huge it is broken down into ten divisions dealing with separate disease categories. Congress says NIH has "brought into being the most productive scientific community centered upon health and disease that the world has ever known."

To NIH the Congress now allots about $1.25 billion a year, compared to about $890 million for medical research given all other federal departments. Industry adds about $890 million yearly to health R & D and all other private sources close to $120 million, making up the $3.3 billion total.

The National Institutes of Health follow a firm policy of deliberately shying away from managing or directing the extramural research projects they support. The NIH open-door policy was designed to encourage any fresh new idea that might one day improve the nation's health posture.

Such a promising fresh idea was hyperbaric medicine when it burst anew on the American scene in the early 1960s.

Overnight came an explosion of interest. Doctors in a dozen American medical centers, impressed and inspired by the triumphs of Boerama in Amsterdam, immediately clamored for chambers and research grants.

On the business side, major fabricators of large size pressure chambers and compressed gas suppliers foresaw help for mankind in the prospect of a new source of corporate profit. The NIH lent an attentive ear to the aggressive and imaginative segment of the medical world eager to get cranked up in HBO and universities and teaching hospitals. Congress got interested, too.

However, the uproar over this new therapy caused frowns in another sector of Washington, the quasi-official National Academy of Sciences-National research Council, the independent agency chartered in 1863 by Congress and President Lincoln as advisor to the federal government on any question of science or technology.

Scientists high in the NAS-NRC recalled the previous fizzle of high-pressure oxygenation therapy. Had the situation changed substantially from the past? Were there truly bright prospects that HBO could be a useful medical tool? The National Academy decided to summon a blue-ribbon panel of experts to try to provide clear-cut answers.

This NAS-NRC ad hoc committee went to Washington in 1962 for a series of workshop sessions. The nine scientists spent many days digging into every aspect of HBO in utmost detail and sifting the positive and negative factors. The following spring, they produce their classic government white paper, a 14,000 word report titled: "Hyperbaric Oxygenation: Potentialities and Problems."

The report concluded that indeed there was a need an opportunity for research in this field, but urged that investigators move with caution because oxygen under pressure could be dangerous and tricky.

Scientists should take another hard look at what was then known of the physiology of oxygen transport and utilization, the white paper suggested, in conjunction with controlled and integrated study of the limitations and possible benefits to be expected in a number of abnormal states. Singled out were pulmonary or cardiovascular insufficiency or anomaly, anaerobic infections, malignancy, poisoning, traumatic ischemia, and shock.

The report reminded prospective HBO investigators that they would find useful the one hundred years' experience of caisson and tunnel workers in compressed air, as well as the US Navy's diving history which had developed parameters of depths, exposure times, oxygen tolerance, and recompression procedures in accidental decompression sickness.

These fields of activity, said the ad hoc committee, provided a valuable but limited background on which to base studies of the physiological effects, limitations, hazards and possible clinical applications of hyperbaric oxygenation. Early clinical reports from Europe and initial experimental studies in this country supported the likelihood that the modality would be of therapeutic importance. Still, said the report, the fundamental information needed to prove its value was not yet available.

Adequate and safe chambers for animal and human pressurization would be costly, cumbersome, and hazardous. The tank designs current in 1962-63 should be regarded only as pilot plants, pending identification of the ultimate role of HBO as a laboratory investigative tool or an adjunct to the clinical armamentarium.

The report also strongly urged the US medical profession to devote a concentrated effort to control basic studies on animals and humans, adding:

"It is recommended that initially the number of hyperbaric facilities, especially those designed for human research, be limited to those where qualified teams of scientists at university or university-caliber medical research centers are supported by fully adequate facilities, continued funding and specialized technical personnel."

In their wisdom a decade ago, the NAS-NRC experts foresaw the imperative need for some central guidance in hyperbaric development and warned against a breakdown in open communication between the scattered, and often rival, investigators. Citing the desirability of some control agency, the white paper said success in such a function would permit more rapid accumulation and evaluation of clinical experience, help eliminate unnecessary duplication of effort, and foster widespread application of the best therapeutic and research techniques.

A major worry to the NAS-NRC panel was the mystery of man's easy vulnerability to being poisoned by the very drug—oxygen—which was the keystone of the therapy.

Their report cautioned sternly that experimenters were immediately confronted with the physiological limitations of oxygen toxicity, terming this a sovereign consideration, since there might well be a narrow margin between therapeutic effects and unacceptable transient or lasting tissue damage to the retina, lungs, or central nervous system.

So little was known about the mechanism of such damage and the limits of tolerance were so inadequately defined, full realization of the potential benefits of hyperbaric oxygenation would depend upon the extent to which oxygen toxicity can be circumvented.

The white paper warned that patients and attendants alike are subjected to the hazards of fire, explosion, decompression sickness, gas embolism, toxic fumes and the discomforts of barotitus (inner ear squeeze) and barosinusitis (similar pain in the paranasal sinuses).

Despite this admonitory tone, the report was not trying to scare off investigators. For the next paragraph read:

"With dual regard to the hazards involved, there is apparent justification for the current enthusiasm. Basic equipment is available and physical safeguards are adequately prescribed..."

The report proposed some specific research priorities. Mentioned were refinement of methods of measuring tissue oxygenation, the relationship between oxygen delivery and cellular oxygenation, the role of hypothermia (body cooling), the effects of hyperbaric oxygenation on the actions of gaseous or volatile anesthetic agents, the interaction of drugs with high-pressure oxygen, the mechanisms of variations and limits of oxygen tolerance, means of early detection of harmful effects of oxygen, and the testing of multiple inert-gas mixtures in decompression studies.

The authors of "Hyperbaric Oxygenation: Potentialities and Problems" did their chore thoroughly, but when they grappled with the complex reaction of the human body to the simple act of taking a breath, they could only confess that indeed there are great physiological mysteries for which we desperately need helpful answers. As they put it:

"The complex mechanism of oxygen transport from the pulmonary alveolus to its ultimate destination in the mitochondrion is basic to life in the mammalian organism... In Haldane's words, 'Oxygen lack not only stops the machine but also wrecks the machinery.'"

They were pointing up the multitude of complications that can transcend the orderly business of our circulating blood gathering its load of oxygen in the lungs (pulmonary alveolus) and routinely carrying it to the energy elements in the individual cell (mitochondria). That movement can be successfully monitored; but when the oxygen reaches its final destination within the tiny cell and is absorbed by that energy element in the cytoplasm, the sharpest eyes of medical science can't keep track of it.

Tiny glass needles are being drawn finer and finer to serve as probes, but none is yet minute enough to invade an individual cell and take a reading on its precise oxygen tension, how much has actually diffused from the blood.

Why the reading from an individual cell warrant such importance was spelled out in the white paper:

"Diffusion characteristics are surely modified when metabolizing cells are part of the diffusion path. One of the most crucial unanswered questions in the hyperbaric field is the extent to which ischemic (oxygen starved) tissues can derive oxygen by diffusion from a neighboring area having normal blood supply. At least one line of reasoning suggests a very disappointing conclusion: the length of normal capillaries may not exceed one millimeter (slightly less than the thickness of a dime), yet in this short distance the oxygen tension of normally flowing blood can apparently drop almost 2,000 millimeters of mercury as dissolved oxygen is removed. It is reasonable then to suppose that the oxygen tension could drop to zero in less than one millimeter of radial distance through metabolizing cells even if oxygen tension in the capillary were exceptionally high. The value of HBO may thus be negligible if an area of complete ischemia exceeds a millimeter or two in any dimension. Present methods of determining tissue oxygen tension are not adequate to provide reliable ancestry to questions such as these."

The point the ad hoc committee sought to make was simply that much more is required for healthy functioning of an individual cell than adequate oxygen. The cell must, for instance, receive nutrients from the blood. The debris of metabolism must be carried away; especially critical is the carbon dioxide content. It would be difficult to imagine a more complex, delicate, and fragile balance than that needed in an individual cell, one of the utter millions in our bodies.

The report dramatized the ambiguities of human physiology by pointing out that the peculiarities of supplying oxygen in physical solution at high oxygen tension include the possibility that cells at the arterial end of a capillary may be poisoned by oxygen while others less than a millimeter away are dying of hypoxia (oxygen starvation). The prestigious National Academy of Sciences-National Research Council had tacitly elevated hyperbaric oxygenation to a high research level by deeming it worthy of a full-scale government white paper. Curiously, this extraordinary move to produce an excellent blueprint for development never made much of an impression. Medical journals and hospital and pharmaceutical magazines published summaries, but the text was not widely circulated.

More importantly, the suggestions and guidelines that could have provided orderly pursuit of HBO research were generally ignored, if read at all. Most investigators, it turned out, were single-minded individuals who took pretty much at face value the government's precepts against bureaucratic interference. Once they had federal grants in hand, these experimenters chose their own paths and timetables for testing whatever idea had come to mind.

This suited the National Institutes of Health whose director (until early 1973), Dr. Robert Q. Marston, had assured Congress that real scientific progress will come through "using the collective wisdom of the expert scientists and clinicians working in the field to determine what should be done and how it should be done."

Marston reiterated in 1971 to a House Appropriation Subcommittee his hands off-policy. NIH, he testified, viewed the role of the federal government in biomedical research as one of stimulating, assisting, and supporting competent investigators rather than one of directing or managing them.

If there was any national traffic cop regulating the flow of medical research spending, he would have to exist within the National Institutes of Health. Yet he would be a composite of outside scientists, rather than a bureaucratic insider.

Marston explained to Congress that NIH believed the primary support mechanism for biomedical research was grants-in-aid to permit a competent investigator to do what he believed possible, necessary, and productive. To judge whether the grant applicant was indeed competent and whether his proposed project was sufficiently worthwhile to merit investing public funds in its support, NIH had set up over the years an elaborate system of review groups, known as study sections.

There were about fifty of these, covering every scientific discipline and clinical field with which NIH was concerned; with members drawn from among leaders in each of these disciplines and fields.

Marston testified that this peer review system had played a vital part in making NIH extramural programs responsive to the opportunities for progress and to the needs of the biomedical research community. In his view, it had preserved the intellectual freedom of scientists and clinicians while getting them involved in research of national importance.

Any hyperbaric experimenter savvy enough to know how the government plays their game lost no time in getting in line at NIH. In 1963 the first three grants-in-aid were made for HBO projects. It was a small beginning, totaling only $54,300 for the year, but the field was so hot everybody expected a lot more federal financial support.

And it did come.

During the ten years ending in 1972, the National Institutes of Health put a total of $5.3 billion into 129,000 research projects of all kinds. Of that bounty, HBO got $7.5 million to finance 193 projects, comparatively a mere drop in the bucket.

It is significant, however, that specific hyperbaric research grants proliferated quickly and reached the level of $1 million dollars a year in 1969 and have pretty well stayed above that mark since. Also, an additional $500,000 year is being granted to studies on oxygen toxicity.

Unfortunately, the most helpful recommendations of the white paper were ignored. No central agency was established to call signals. Perhaps setting up one would have been impossible. In our free society any persuasive physician with a sudden hankering to become a hyperbarist could order up a tank as long as he could somehow wheedle the price. No government license or approval was required.

In the first hectic months of 1962-63, it seemed that the stunning news coming across the Atlantic from Amsterdam had triggered a kind of national derby among America's big hospitals to see which would be the first to establish its own Hyperbaric Department.

Then hospital administrators suddenly paused and pondered the initial cost of the sophisticated hardware as well as the operational expense—an estimated \$40,000 to \$100,000 a year for personnel to keep the chamber on 24-hour standby. Most of them cooled off.

Experimental therapy began helter-skelter. In retrospect many of the initial protocols seem poorly designed or tended to waste their main thrust on problems that had been previously examined.

The initial harvest of such an impetuous and badly organized beginning could only be a confusing mixture of meager success and astounding disappointment, the latter with occasional chilling consequences.

Even the National Academy of Science-National Research Council began to lose interest. It made no follow-up on its recommendations for a central agency or an information exchange, and within five years half the experts who wrote its white paper had become inactive in the field.

The academy did try to foster interest by joining with NIH to provide a substantial fund to underwrite the Third International Symposium on Hyperbaric Medicine in 1965 at Duke University Medical Center, and subsidized publication of those proceedings, a fifteen-dollar-book which was fairly well distributed to US medical libraries.

By the mid-1960s any big push to interest Washington in hyperbaric research had passed its zenith, and that was just as well. Congress had suddenly gotten hot, along with President Nixon, in declaring war on the big killers—cancer, plus diseases of the heart, lung, and blood vessels. More millions were shoveled into NIH with the idea that enough money would surely make it possible to find the cures that could extend American life expectancy and avert the yearly multi-million dollar drain in lost productivity and doctor-hospital bills.

A series of interviews in 1972 with key members and staff directors of the committees on health in both the Senate and House disclosed that hyperbaric research had practically no priority rating with Congress.

It seemed unlikely that Chairman Edward Kennedy's (D., Massachusetts) Senate subcommittee of Health could work for months shaping up its 1.3 billion more on heart-lung diseases without somehow touching on hyperoxygenation, which is so interlinked with cardiovascular physiology. Yet Kennedy could recall no mention. The staff director, Leroy G. Goldman, went even further; he didn't believe any hyperbaric legislation had ever been brought before the subcommittee.

In the House, the Interstate and Foreign Commerce Committee, which initiates health legislation, was concerned in 1972 about medical researchers' competition for the federal dollar. Jim Menger, a top committee aide for twenty years, said committee members recognized the merit of hyperbaric therapy.

"But," Menger told an interviewer, "if we could take the money that's spent on hyperbaric operating chambers and spend it immunizing kids against rubella (also known as German Measles), we'd accomplished a hell of a lot more for public health."

The 1,650 page transcript of the House Appropriations Subcommittee hearings in 1971 on the NIH budget, which covered the entire range of government-sponsored medical research, makes only one mention of hyperbaric medicine, it is very brief.

The director of the Child Health and Human Development Institute, Dr. Gerald D. LaVeck, was being questioned about senility research:

Rep. Robert H. Michel (R., Illinois): "You mentioned the use of high pressure oxygen for the treatment of impaired mental function in old age. What will be your support level in fiscal 1973 and can you estimate how long it is going to take before you can tell if this treatment has a value?"

Dr. LaVeck: "We are supporting two studies, one at the State University of New York at Buffalo and one at Duke University to determine the value of this treatment. The cost is $74,000 for fiscal year 1972 and estimated at $74,000 for fiscal 1973. I think within the next year or two we should know if this technique has promise."

It is rather startling to find this brief item the only mention of HBO that appears in about three-quarters of a million words of testimony intended to cover the whole spectrum of the most promising avenues open in medical researchers.

By coincidence the chairman of the Senate State labor and Public Welfare committee, whose umbrella authority covers the subcommittee of health, is quite knowledgeable about HBO, and personally alert to its potential. He is Senator Harrison A. Williams, Jr., brisk, mid-fiftyish Democrat from New Jersey who was a Navy pilot and a lawyer.

My research indicated that Williams had taken dives at Saint Barnabas Medical Center in his home state. But during an interview he explained he had entered Saint Barnabas in February 1971 for conventional treatment of cellulitis (a skin inflammation) on his leg and visited the hyperbaric department out of curiosity and learned much about it.

Williams, turning the tables on the interviewer and firing questions of his own, seemed surprised by the large number of diseases which have responded to HBO. He was especially interested in the experiments aimed at reversing senility.

"Well, it's never been thoroughly researched, you see. I'll have to be honest with you, at this point it's a low priority. There's no kidding around here, we have not been able to—there's a bureaucratic negative. Gee whiz, it was like a swamp owl, the bigger and brighter the light you put it in their face, the blinder they get. It could have high priority with me, but I don't know where in the hell we are going."

During discussion of the clinical work at Saint Barnabas, Williams disclosed that he planned to take his mother, 81 years old, there for about three weeks of treatment. He described her as physically pretty sturdy and said her memory was not bad just "annoying."

The senator also was trying to work out his own schedule so he could go to St. Barnabas on weekends and take dives in the chamber, in an admittedly hit-skip version of the executive brush-up.

Williams was interested in Hart's work at Long Beach Naval Hospital and especially liked the suggestion that the Navy surgeon would make an excellent witness if the Senate ever studied the use of HBO to relieve memory loss in old people.

If senility studies across the country develop more convincing evidence, HBO might get a break again in Washington. Senator Williams has great influence, of course, in the special Senate subcommittee on aging, and was considering the possibility of holding hearings on the potential of HBO.

What is the current attitude of the NAS-NRC toward HBO? In 1970, the academy formed its own Institute of Medicine, headed by Dr. John Hogness, former dean of the University of Washington School of Medicine. The announced purpose of the Institute of medicine is to "... identify, for study and analysis, important issues and problems that relate to health and medicine; prepare authoritative statements on these issues and problems when, in the judgment of the Institute, such statements would be in the public interest; initiate and conduct studies of national policy and planning for healthcare and health-related education and research... and disseminate information to the public..."

Currently, Hogness explained that there was no special concern about the status of hyperbaric research. The Institute was looking into an allied field, the ability of man to stay submerged in an undersea habitat for weeks at a time in offshore oil drilling and exploration. This work might possibly shed some light on oxygen or pressure tolerances similar to those required in a hyperbaric chamber.

Such negative overtones do not obscure the presence of significant fresh interest in clinical application of hyperbaric therapy.

Despite a general slump in the sale of big chambers, one fabricator, Vacudyne of Chicago, added a big new medical center opening in 1972 to its roster of hyperbaric customers. The new Nassau County Medical Center at East Meadow, Long Island, New York, was installing a 100,000 dollar chamber in its nineteen-story Hospital.

Likewise, the Navy was taking bids on a three-chamber complex at its New London, Connecticut, submarine medicine center. The price tag was estimated at $750,000.

Worldwide interest also remained high enough to warrant scheduling the Fifth International Hyperbaric Congress for August 1973 at Vancouver, British Columbia, Canada.

The conference president, Dr. W. G. Trap, anticipated 300 delegates, mostly physicians from the United States but about thirty from Japan and a similar number from Britain, others from France, Australia, New Zealand, Italy, Germany, and a few from Russia, Czechoslovakia, and Romania.

15

THE EXPERTS SEARCH FOR ANSWERS

Considering all pros and cons, what is the best judgment of top experts on where hyperbaric medicine actually stands today? Are they in agreement on precisely which disease and trauma conditions the tank treatments definitely can control or cure? Do they share a common view on the quirky hazards which sometimes bedevil exposure to oxygen, and agree on how best to guard against poisoning their patients? What do they expect of the future?

An authoritative summation and appraisal of such pertinent questions would go far toward unscrambling the jumbled picture of HBO which now confronts not only the uninitiated layman but also most general practice doctors.

Those obviously best qualified to pass such judgment are the several hundred medical scientists who were drawn as pioneers in the early 1960s into America's rebirth of interest in pressure oxygenation. These physicians, surgeons, radiologists, anesthesiologists, biochemists, psychiatrists, and psychologists scattered all across the country have spent a full decade now literally on the inside of the research and clinical development of this therapy.

Unfortunately, they are not of one mind: far from it.

They are in a serious way split on fundamentals, all the way down to the most nitty-gritty question of all: whether HBO offers enough beneficial results to compensate for the risk associated with its use.

The experts fall generally into two opposing camps, but also splinter into sub-cliques which wrangle on four or five side issues. Some disagreements run deep and wide.

While this discord tends to hamstring the advance of hyperbaric medicine, such confusion really should not be much surprise. The differing attitudes and opinions of each pioneer experimenter largely have taken shape from this individual research and clinical experience. These results have been, of course, astoundingly varied. The range goes from ignominious flops to thrilling triumphs, middled by lots of inconclusive work.

Most of it was tough going, and the experimenting took a visible toll.

Some of those who rushed eagerly and aggressively into HBO therapy candidly concede that ten years of often quixotic ups and downs have stung their faith and dampened their ardor. A handful became totally disillusioned and quit altogether. Others paused to take a second look and decided to slow down, relegating once-ambitious studies to the backburners of their imaginations.

However, the majority of those who most vigorously explored this old-new medical frontier throughout the 1960s indicate they will press on, in one way or another, in hope of eventually achieving the unqualified acceptance that has flirted with and eluded HBO for three centuries.

The obvious consequence of the absence of any expert consensus, or top-level guideline, is that the public is still left to pretty much make up its own mind.

The problems that create conflict among the experts have been examined in earlier chapters. Perhaps the most overriding debate is whether tank therapy has cleared all hurdles and is ready for widespread use in all hospitals or should be severely restricted to research-oriented centers and limited to further experimental studies.

Duke University Medical Center's Herbert Saltzman, a renowned authority, says bluntly it still is too risky for general use in hospitals at the community level. Boston's William Bernhard, who made history with America's first HBO blue-baby surgery, has come around to the same way of thinking. Hyperbaric chambers, Bernhard asserts, are inherently expensive and dangerous and should not be available in the country as a whole.

These by no means are isolated negative voices, several other HBO authorities regard oxygen chambers with a very cautious if not outright jaundiced eye. However, such extremism quite obviously runs counter to a more sizable body of positive feeling, the proof of which is convincingly demonstrated by the presence of active hyperbaric chambers in scores of cities all across the United States, including a sizable number in small community hospitals.

Still the range of thumbs-down feeling is broad. For example, Claude Hitchcock, who snared for Minneapolis in 1963 one of the nation's largest and most expensive chamber complexes, is not quite so disillusioned as Saltzmann and Bernard. But he has decided HBO is too limited to be the great boon he envisioned ten years ago; although he believes still it deserves a definite role in the total over-all medical picture.

Top physiologist Edward Lanphier calls it a bandwagon that turned into a pumpkin. That doesn't mean he has abandoned the field. On more than one occasion he has willingly crawled out of bed at midnight to open up his research chamber at State University of New York at Buffalo to handle an emergency case. He never had any doubt he could help; and in one instance saved the life of a Canadian driver stricken by the bends. He favors more research.

Over and over in my interviews with a hundred principal hyperbaric clinicians and researchers the dialogue raised and underscored one vulnerability—the uncertainty of the sometime medical miracle.

Even the best documented life-saving triumphs credited to the tank—such as the Sandra Olsons, the Corporal Helfers, the Beverly Kreuters—are challenged by some skeptics. How, they ask, could these recoveries be ascribed solely to hyperoxygenation? It is not uncommon, they argue, to frequently encounter inexplicable instances of so-called miracle cures—curious cases where the doctors give up and the patient recovers in spite of everything.

A George Hart might shoot down such a challenge with a succinct reminder that Corporal Helfer had been declining for months, every other known treatment had been tried and still a young Marine was "going down the tubes"—literally wasting away and certainly dying before the doctors' eyes until the tank brought him back. And the medical logs verify thousands of similar successes.

The second challenge raised by doubting doctors is much tougher. They primarily are interested in knowing that beyond doubt HBO treatments will produce consistently beneficial results every time in every patient. That, they contend, is the true test of effective therapy. And, considering all aspects of difficulties of tank treatments, if they can have that specific assurance, why bother?

That kind of rock hard evidence is simply not available. Not everybody responds to oxygenation in precisely the same fashion, as explained earlier, principally because of the enormous range of variables possible within man's complex physiologic mechanism that regulates oxygen uptake and blood circulation.

And it is the absence of that precise guarantee that accentuates the most talked about fear in hyperbaric medicine—oxygen poisoning. There seems no likelihood of any great forward stride for this modality until a better understanding is gained of oxygen toxicity. How this poison condition arises is a many-faceted mystery that continues to baffle the best minds in medical research. The puzzle will not be solved overnight.

A layman picking through case histories of the thousands of desperately sick people reported substantially helped by tank treatment feels that this hazard may be magnified out of proportion by ultra -cautious investigators. To him it might seem a potential yet fairly infrequent danger to patients, one which the fully experienced HBO technician could intercept and thus prevent any disruption of safe therapy.

Buffalo's Harry Alvis supports such a view. Oxygen toxicity, he says bluntly, becomes a problem only to the uninformed and inexperienced. He knows a lot about the subject. As editor of the hyperbaric medicine newsletter, he maintains an excellent overview of what's taking place in the field. And his extensive clinical experience is predated by a long career as a Navy submarine and diving medical office officer where he was regularly involved in pressure oxygenation.

Alvis's rule is to keep Hyperbaric therapy within reasonable limits. By that he means intermittent exposures at pressures of 2.5 to 3 ATA lasting no longer than 90 to 120 minutes.

In no way does he attempt to minimize the destructive force that can be unleashed by careless or reckless use of a chamber. The same kind of risk is involved in driving an automobile, Alvis points out; a motorist's safety depends on his experience and knowledgeability of his equipment and using it in a safe and sane manner.

Dr. Charles Billings, who operates a research chamber at Ohio State University in Columbus as professor of environmental medicine, sites fire in drawing a similar analogy. He points out that fire can be used to heat a home or make a jet plane go or it can destroy you. It's all in how you handle it; and he feels the same is true of hyperbaric oxygen.

Despite reassuring talk about experience and knowledgeability, many researchers steadfastly harbor grave concern. True accurate guidelines have been established to keep pressure and length of dives with acceptable safe limits. But one points out, these schedules were developed over the years from experience with normal people, primarily healthy young Navy divers. In contrast, clinical hyperbarists cope primarily with desperately ill people of all ages who do not necessarily respond to standard physiologic norms because of their disease. The facial twitching and other signs that foretell the onset of convulsions usually give ample warning. Thus alerted, the hyperbaric doctor usually can prevent or quickly terminate such a seizure by shutting off the flow of 100% oxygen to his patient. But several experts fear unseen damaging effects on the central nervous system that may not show up until years later.

Duke's Saltzman concedes there are valid indications for use of hyperbaric therapy and that there will be more, not fewer, in the coming decade. At the same time, he doesn't retreat at all from his opinion that not enough research has been done to justify its general use. He is adamant that the toxicity puzzle must first be solved.

It would be deceptive oversimplification to try to array hyperbarists against each other under good guys and bad guys labels. Too narrow a focus can miss the fact that the danger of poisoning patients with oxygen is not limited to hyperbarists alone but is genuinely feared by all doctors who put their patients on oxygen.

As Minneapolis's Hitchcock points out, oxygen toxicity is a very real threat in every hospital in the world where respirator support is used and the patient is given anything more than the 20% oxygen, the equivalent of normal room air. To illustrate, Hitchcock mentions three typical kinds of cases likely to get respirator support: surgical patients in the recovery room, and auto-accident casualty with a damaged lung, or a newborn baby with hyaline membrane disease or other pulmonary distress.

Any of these, says Hitchcock, kept breathing 60 to 80% oxygen for longer than four or five days is in critical danger of becoming toxic. Other physicians talk about hospital oxygen used too long, hastening death.

Ohio State's Billings agrees with Hitchcock and says that harmful overuse of oxygen doubtless is more common than realized.

He likens oxygen to a two-edged sword, both sides equally sharp, with considerable advantages and liabilities.

Some HBO studies have turned out as flops, in his view, because of failure of the experimenters to fully appreciate the physiological aberrations that can be induced by hyperoxygenation.

Doctors seeking to achieve one effect may get exactly the opposite, harming the patient. He feels this can occur in instances where there is specific reaction between high pressure oxygen and low or normal carbon dioxide tension in the blood. Instead of the desired hyperoxia or oxygen drenching, the treatment may produce a degree of hypoxia, or oxygen starvation.

While the toxicity hazard possibly is HBO's biggest bugaboo, it certainly does not deserve total blame for any lack of progress. Sharp criticism frequently is directed at early advocates for their eagerness and haste and heavy-handed recklessness.

Alan Thal, who was chairman of the National Academy of Sciences white paper committee, partially attributes the current setback to "overenthusiasm" generated in the early 1960s. That opinion is echoed by Buffalo's Alvis. In three or four places, says Alvis, people went into it too big. He asserts: "Probably this overkill aspect is what did it more harm than anything else."

Despite all that, Elvis still strongly there is a place for HBO treatments in the overall armamentarium of the medical profession.

Unfortunately, he laments, to go first-class in the field is very expensive and installations cannot be made to pay their way unless, as he puts it, "they are simply exploited." Alvis sees that as a constant temptation where the Investment is large.

No one has yet defected from the hyperbaric leader ranks with a more surprising jolt than Minneapolis's Hitchcock. The change-about dismayed his colleagues in the field, and with good reason. Hitchcock had been one of the first in America to see promise in tank therapy; eager and aggressive, he had acquired a costly multi-chamber complex specifically designed for surgery. But in eight years he went from red hot to ice cold.

His disenchantment first surfaced at the January 1970 First Western Conference on Hyperbaric Medicine at Los Angeles. Hitchcock's blunt negativism caught fellow delegates by surprise, and nettled or angered many. When the Minneapolis surgeon got up to speak, he said simply he no longer believed that HBO had any substantial benefits that couldn't be provided by other treatments, unless possibly in dealing with infections. Even that effect, he said, was dubious.

At once a verbal storm erupted. Several leading investigators were on their feet to take him on. Cowley of Baltimore expressed amazement that Hitchcock no longer felt as so many did that HBO should be used in all gas-gangrene cases but merely in selected instances and only after surgical debridement, which would invalidate the primary advantage of hyperoxygenation. The Minneapolis surgeon would not back down. His reply to Cowley was that he had treated enough gas gangrene both in and out of the tank to know what worked best.

Gangrene was not the only topic that provoked quarrels. When Hart advised the conference about his amazing success in healing burns in his tanks at Long Beach neighborhood Hospital, Hitchcock countered that "burns can be nicely controlled with silver nitrate," saying the tank was not needed.

The surgeon from Minneapolis wrangled with his peers that day on so many points that Jacobson of New York's Mount Sinai Hospital finally snapped that Hitchcock's devastating critique is "pure hogwash."

And Trapp, who directs the hyperbaric program at the University of British Columbia in Vancouver, deplored Hitchcock's "tragic" attitude.

On a milder scale, the same kind of controversy has also emerged in subsequent conferences. For instance, at the 1972 Norwalk, Connecticut Symposium, three or four doctors strongly challenged each other's views. They were chiefly at odds over the advisability of using HBO to combat the myocardial infarction which results from coronary heart attacks, and on potential hazards associated with putting any patient with viremia, any virus in the blood, in the chamber. Hart thought that extremely risky.

The Western Conference uproar spawned the false impression that Hitchcock was abandoning all his oxygen work and closing down his beautiful tanks. He did not quit. He has drastically reduced his chamber use, though; in 1972 he averaged just about one hyperbaric patient a month. He continues selective treatment in his chamber of gas gangrene, estimating that he oxygenates about one of three. Some of his research funding which substantially financed the heavy cost of operating the complex ran out in 1972 and Hitchcock got busy trying to devise appealing new studies for using his chambers.

In light of his strong negative outburst, Hitchcock was asked toward the end of 1972 for his current assessment of the value of the hyperbaric treatment.

It was by no means as glum as those who listen to him at the Western Conference might expect. Hitchcock now says he would personally like to always have a chamber available as long as his hospital is called on to be a center of referral cases of the bends, carbon monoxide poisoning, and gas gangrene. (Patients have been sent to his tanks from as far as Kansas City.) And he thinks it is reasonable to have hyperbaric facilities available to the public in various parts of the country for these services alone.

Far less favorable is the present attitude of blue-baby surgeon Bernhard.

His enthusiasm took a jarring fall after his initial success in salvaging infants with congenital heart defects in the old Harvard tank earned him a magnificent government built multi-chamber complex. But that costly facility is now only used about seventy-five times a year, and Bernhard's team needs it for only about 10% of their blue-baby surgery.

It just wasn't the real answer for the difficulties of that kind of operation, Bernhard decided. He thinks an improved heart-lung device will offer the surgeon more freedom and the tiny patient more support. In addition, he now believes hyperbaric treatments are not only dangerous because of the toxicity threat but otherwise of limited usefulness.

Bernhard considers only three clinical areas as "possible targets": (1) extensive gas-gangrene infections, (2) carbon monoxide intoxication, and (3) as a surgical adjunct and occasional blue-baby operations.

These are limited targets, Bernhard contends, because gas gangrene and carbon monoxide poisoning are "quite rare" in the United States. Other hyperbarists will give him an argument on that; several HBO departments log in a substantial number of both types of cases every year. Bernhard seems to be basing his evaluation on the fact that his tanks get only about one gas-gangrene patient a year.

However, just one of the chambers in Buffalo, at Millard Fillmore Hospital, treats about five times that number, handling forty gas gangrene cases between 1964 and 1972. Likewise, tank treatment for carbon monoxide poisoning certainly is not rare in cities like Milwaukee where Kindwall's educational program has alerted ambulance and fire rescue squads to the tank's availability.

Elaborating on his second thoughts, Bernhard feels that enthusiasm for hyperbaric medicine has far outdistanced its clinical and research usefulness "up to this moment." He can't think of even one additional "solid clinical indication" for the therapy.

That is precisely the reason Saltsman considers it more important to work now on gaining fundamental knowledge—for instance, the actual mechanisms of the human lung—than to worry about the specific roadblocks delaying HBO's advance such as toxicity and the body's inability to transport oxygen to critical tissue areas when blood circulation is impaired.

"All those negative results" of the twelve to fourteen years since the start of the combined British-Dutch efforts, he says," must be telling us something—either that the system lacks merit as a therapeutic modality or that information was not available to help doctors apply the modality successfully." Saltzman thinks it is the second position.

The Duke experimenter concedes there is some rationale for benefit in hyperbaric treatment, but he fears the uplift most patients get from the treatment can lead to an artificial evaluation.

What is needed, Saltzmann feels, is actual life-or-death evidence. For illustration he uses the example of a patient dying of refractory leukemia. If he were given hyperbaric treatment and got well, Saltzman would consider that an important measurement because it would differ from all past experience. On the other hand, if HBO is used on a patient who feels pain in his foot when he walks because of poor circulation and afterward says he feels better, "you haven't really learned anything."

The real test is how the long-term course of the disease is affected, he says, contending that that judgment can't be made by simply putting people in chambers. He feels doctors might learn something in 10 or 15 years of doing that, but it's a very inefficient way of going about it, "and the answers could still be wrong."

Viewing the problem as a realist, Saltzman concedes it is probably true that sick people in many parts of the country are now denied the opportunity to receive hyperbaric treatment because the public is so much in the dark about it.

Unfortunately, Saltzman laments, the lack of communication in medicine is not limited to hyperbaric oxygen but exists at all levels and affects almost all medical problems. There really is no good reverse distribution system for medical care in effect, in other words a way of getting out new information at the right time. Salzman says there probably is no realistic way of doing that for all medical problems because it would require, in his opinion, making physicians out of everyone.

His answer to the situation is to have people at primary medical care areas who know where to turn when these questions arise.

Like others an organized medicine, Saltzman fears unscrupulous physicians may attempt to exploit hyperbaric therapy for easy profit. Alvis also considers that a distinct threat, which would be utterly ruinous. Across the Atlantic, Boerema also worries about that, asserting something akin to quackery killed HBO's mid-nineteenth-century boom and warning:

"The danger is menacing now... I received a large number of letters from different countries in which doctors as well as layman asked me to put patients in the chamber for reasons which were quite irrational and sometimes even ridiculous...The opportunity for big money-making is present. This would mean the end of this therapy."

Any attempt to forecast today how hyperbaric medicine's future will evolve would have to employ a lot of guesswork. An enormous amount of research is going on in all phases of medicine, many projects pinpointing directly on oxygen use under pressure, and thousands of studies dealing with heart, lung, blood circulation, and the like which could have an intimate bearing on respiration.

Laboratory studies tend to percolate rather slowly; it may take years to achieve a means of short-circuiting oxygen toxicity. Some heartening signs of success, though, are peeking through. The method of avoiding the hazard might be as simple as giving the patient a pill before he takes his dive.

Dr. Aaron P. Sanders and Associates of Saltzman's at Duke ran studies on animals which were given a combination of standard anticonvulsant drugs such as those epileptics take to ward off impending seizures and a rather ordinary chemical, sodium succinate. This medication seemed to lessen the poisonous effect of the high oxygen doses on the guinea pig; but a side effect was that effectiveness of the oxygenation seem to be less, too.

At the University of Kansas School of Pharmacy, Dr. Morris D. Faiman found that disulfiram (the Antabuse that gives alcoholics such a nasty reaction that they don't dare drink while taking it) and its chemical relative, Diethyldithiocarbamate, protected mice from oxygen poisoning, even under 6 ATA, for six hours.

Ironically, the search for the answer to the riddle of oxygen toxicity will get important help from Navy experiments aimed at sending an unarmored diver a mile deep into the sea, where water pressure would crush a conventional submarine as easily as an eggshell.

So that scientists can simulate such a dive on land, the world's strongest hyperbaric chamber has been built at State University of New York at Buffalo. The super super tank, 8 by 22 feet, has five-inch thick steel walls and can be pressurized to 170 ATA, or 2,500 pounds per square inch. That equals ocean pressure at 5600 feet, more than five times as deep as a diver has descended.

In the Buffalo tests, divers breathe the exotic mixtures of oxygen and helium or other rare gases. High among the thousands of questions to be answered is precisely how divers tolerate oxygen under extremes of pressure and duration. The experiments, directed by Lanphier, may have no clear-cut application to clinical hyperbaric medicine because on their simulated deep plunge, the divers will be breathing not even normal room air, but perhaps as little as 1% oxygen mixed with other gases.

However, the physiologic secrets of respiration must be enormously explored to achieve mile- deep dives; and those studies surely will give a better understanding of oxygen within the body.

A simulated dive to 1,000 feet already has been made in a smaller "wet pot" at Duke's hyperbaric complex, a little short of the French record descent of 1,190 feet in 1968. The deep dive experiments also will give better guidelines on the critical decompression schedules that are now a worry to clinicians. The almost universally used US Navy decompression tables are just good guesstimates when applied to many patients, especially the febrile elderly, because the schedules are based on Navy divers in good condition.

Something that sounds like a product of science fiction, "fluid breathing," also is being investigated. If human lungs, like a fish's gills, can breathe an oxygenated liquid instead of a gas mixture, perhaps divers could go to 10,000 feet.

This far-out idea has been successfully tested with animals. Dogs have breathed oxygenated water in laboratory devices for forty-five minutes and mice for up to eighteen hours and have survived. The limiting barrier encountered in the test was not failure to get enough oxygen, but the difficulty of exhausting sufficient carbon dioxide from the lungs.

It would be unusual for fluid breathing to have a direct application to clinical use of HBO, but again the experts feel working toward that eventuality easily could unlock some secret door that now hides the full understanding of the respiration mechanisms.

Doctors would learn much about stroke and senility if they could do the impossible and see inside the human skull so as to measure the amount of precious oxygen the blood delivers to various parts of the brain.

A device to provide that information has been developed by the hyperbaric researchers at New York University. As explained by Theobald Reich and Howard Rusk, 144 semi-conductor radioisotope detectors are arrayed about the head in a mathematical design whose angles were worked out by computer. A technician can set the harmless machine in a couple of minutes. The patient breathes xenon gas through a face mask for one minute. In the lungs, the blood extracts the xenon and circulates it through the body. The detectors trace the xenon entering the brain, and the computer to which they are wired prints out a three-dimensional diagram or picture of detailed blood circulation, something never before achieved.

Previously, Reich explains, there was no way to determine the blood flow in any one loci of the brain; you could only tell in a region. Blood flow could be 100 percent in such a region and zero in another; even angiography doesn't pinpoint precisely what tissue the blood reaches because the dye injected into the arteries thins out, and being diluted, loses its contrast before reaching the small capillaries.

The NYU researchers hope to learn how the blood flow nourishes all the brain substructures, what collateral circulation there is, how the giving of certain drugs may change this distribution of the blood flow. How, for example, not eating cholesterol will reduce the incidence of arterial sclerosis and stroke.

With the machine fully developed, Reich foresees the necessity for five years of human studies to acquire data relating to hyperbaric medicine.

The phrase five years rolls casually off Reich's tongue. In the laboratory-oriented world of painstaking research one year is perhaps equal to a single week in the hurly-burly impatience of ordinary life. Obviously answers to today's urgent questions about Hyperbaric medicine will emerge slowly.

This book has been an attempt to fully explore this little-known field of medicine, to illuminate and ventilate the varied facets of the continuing controversy over its effectiveness and safety, and to indicate its probable future.

As noted, some important researchers believe it is harmful to kindle greater public interest in such an uncertain modality. They contend it is not fully tested and therefore too hazardous for use now in community hospitals.

Yet other competent and equally respected and renowned physicians decry the prevailing ignorance and argue that HBO—even if it is yet an uncertain miracle—has definitely saved thousands of dying patients, and it can save even more lives now!

In this context it is interesting and enlightening to look at the log of one of America's most recently installed units, the Vickers one-patient chamber at Christ Hospital in Cincinnati. In its first year, through November 1972, Cornelia Dettmer compressed the little tank 335 times to treat a total of 42 patients.

One of those was, of course, Beverly Kreuter. It is difficult to see how anyone could blandly characterize the hyperbaric chamber as an unproven research device not yet suitable for use in community hospitals while watching Beverly Kreuter cuddle her twins and exult, "I know it saved my life!"

DIRECTORY OF HYPERBARIC CHAMBERS

IN THE UNITED STATES, CANADA,

MEXICO AND PUERTO RICO

This is the best available state by state listing of shore-based facilities, prepared by the US Navy and brought up to date in early 1973. Although this directory is intended for Navy use, it can be a starting point for anyone inquiring about the availability of HBO therapy in their locality. Obviously, many of the chambers listed here are for research or commercial diving operations, but the personnel in charge should be knowledgeable about the nearest available medical facility.

It is suggested that any communication with any facility listed be directed to "Physician or Officer In Charge, Hyperbaric medicine Department." The Navy, of course, makes no representations about the fitness of any of these chambers or operating personnel. The directory is reprinted with permission of Supervisor of Diving, US Navy, Washington, DC, 20360.

UNITED STATES OF AMERICA

ALABAMA

Redstone Arsenal—Marshall Space Flight Center

ALASKA

Adac—US Naval Station

Kodiak—US Naval Station

CALIFORNIA

Avalon—Avalon Municipal Hospital

Berkeley—White Mountain Laboratory

Coronado—US Navy Underwater Demolition Team 11

Chino—California Institute for Men (prison)

Duarte—City of Hope Medical Center

Edwards Air Force Base—6510th US Air Force Hospital

Goleta—Associated Divers, Inc.

Long Beach—US Naval Shipyard

Long Beach—US Naval Hospital

Los Angeles—Cedars of Lebanon Hospital

Los Angeles—Hospital of the Good Samaritan

Castle Air Force Base—US Air Force 852nd Medical Group

Oakland—Coastal School of Deep Sea Diving

Pacific Grove— Pacific Grove Fire Department

Morris Dam—US Navy Undersea Research

San Clemente Island—US Navy Undersea Research

Point Mugu—Pacific Missile Range

San Diego—US Navy Second Class Diver School

San Diego—US Navy Undersea Research

San Francisco—Presbyterian Pacific Medical Center

San Francisco—Transit Authority Compressed Air Medical Center

San Francisco—Veterans Administration Hospital

San Francisco—Mount Zion Hospital Medical Center

San Francisco—University of California (Beth 307c)

Santa Barbara—California Divers

Santa Barbara—Ocean Systems, Inc.

Santa Barbara—Santa Barbara City College, Marine Technology Program

Santa Ana—US Divers Co.

Vallejo—Mare Island Naval Shipyard

Wilmington—Childers Diving Corporation, Commercial Diving Center

COLORADO

Lowry Air Force Base— US Air Force Dispensary, Physiological Training Unit

Fort Collins—Colorado State University, Department Of Physiology and Biophysics

CONNECTICUT

New London—US Naval Submarine Medical Center

Norwalk—Norwalk Hospital

DISTRICT OF COLUMBIA

Washington—US Navy Experimental Diving Unit

Washington—US Naval Medical Research Institute

Washington—US Naval Oceanographic Office

Washington—US Naval School of Diving And Salvage

FLORIDA

Fort Lauderdale—Divers Training Academy, Inc.

Fort Lauderdale—US Naval Ordinance Lab Test Facility

Gainesville—University Of Florida Shands Teaching Hospital

Kennedy Space Center—John F. Kennedy Space Center

Key West—US Navy Underwater Swimmer School

Leesburg—Lake Community Hospital

Miami—University of Miami School of Marine and Atmospheric Sciences

Panama City—Naval Ship Research and Development Lab

Pensacola—Naval Aerospace Medical Center, Physiological Training Division

GEORGIA

Decatur—Dixie Diving Center

HAWAII

Pearl Harbor—US Naval Base, Explosive Ordnance Disposal Group

Pearl Harbor—US Submarine Base, Fleet Submarine Training Center

Honolulu—University of Hawaii, J. K. K. Look Lab of Oceanographic Engineering

Waimanalo—Makai Undersea Test Range

ILLINOIS

Chicago—Cook County Hospital

Chicago—Edgewater Hospital

Chicago—University of Chicago

Chicago Heights—Saint James Hospital

Park Ridge—Lutheran General Hospital

KANSAS

Kansas City—University of Kansas Medical Center

LOUISIANA

Amelia—S. & H. Subwater Salvage Co., Inc.

Bell Chasse—Action Dives

Bell Chasse—Taylor Diving and Salvage Co., Inc.

Berwick —Fluor Ocean Services, Inc.

Grand Isle—Action Divers

Harvey—Dick Evans, Inc.

Harvey—Pelican Marine Diving Service

Morgan City—Divcon, Inc.

Morgan City—Hydrotech Service, Inc.

Morgan City—Ocean Systems, Inc.

Morgan City—Worldwide Divers, Inc.

New Orleans—Dr. Linwood High Carter, 4343 Elysian Fields Avenue

MARYLAND

Annapolis—Westinghouse Ocean Research and Engineering

Baltimore—University of Maryland School of Medicine

Indian Head—US Naval Ordnance station

Solomons—US Naval Ordinance Lab Test Facility

MASSACHUSETTS
Boston—Boston Children's Hospital Medical Center
Boston—Boston Naval Shipyard
MICHIGAN
Ann Arbor—University of Michigan Medical Center, Underwater Operations Laboratory
Eloise—Wayne County General Hospital
Royal Oak—William Beaumont Hospital
MINNESOTA
Minneapolis—Hennepin County General Hospital
MISSOURI
Kansas City—Saint Luke's Hospital
Saint Louis—McDonnell Douglas Corporation
MONTANA
Fort Peck—US Army Corps of Engineers Headquarters
NEBRASKA
Omaha—University Of Nebraska School of Medicine
NEW HAMPSHIRE
Portsmouth—Portsmouth Naval Shipyard
NEW JERSEY
Hackensack—Hackensack Hospital
Livingston—St. Barnabas Medical Center
Toms River—Ocean County Diving Ltd.
NEW YORK
Buffalo—Millard Fillmore Hospital
Buffalo—Veterans Administration Hospital
Buffalo—State University of New York at Buffalo
Flushing, Long Island—International Underwater Contractors Inc.
New York—Yeshiva University
New York—Montefiore Hospital
New York—Bronx Veterans Administration Hospital

New York—Cornell Medical Center
New York—New York University Medical Center
New York—Mount Sinai Hospital
New York—Columbia Presbyterian Medical Center
NORTH CAROLINA
Durham—Duke University Medical Center
Wilmington—Wrightsville Marine Biomedical Lab
Wilmington-Salem—Bowman Gray School of Medicine
OHIO
Cincinnati—The Christ Hospital
Cleveland—Cleveland Clinic Hospital
Cleveland—Saint Vincent's Charity Hospital
Columbus—Batelle Memorial Institute
Columbus—Ohio State University College of Medicine
Toledo—Medical College of Ohio Hospital
Wright Patterson Air Force Base—US Air Force Medical Center
OKLAHOMA
Oklahoma City—Federal Aviation Administration
OREGON
Oxbow—Idaho Power Co. Oxbow Dam
Portland—Commercial Divers, Inc.
Portland —Fred Devine Diving and Salvage Company, Inc.
PENNSYLVANIA
Allentown—Allentown Osteopathic Hospital
Philadelphia—Hahnemann Medical College
Philadelphia— University of Pennsylvania Medical Center
Philadelphia—Philadelphia Naval Shipyard
Philadelphia—US Naval Base
RHODE ISLAND
Newport—US Naval Base
SOUTH CAROLINA
Beaufort— Marine Corps Air Station

Charleston—US Naval Station
SOUTH DAKOTA
Ellsworth Air Force Base—Physiological Training Unit
Pierre—US Army Corps of Engineers Headquarters
TEXAS
Corpus Christi—Blue Water Industries
Corpus Christi—US Naval Air Station
Dallas—Saint Paul's Hospital
Galveston—University of Texas Medical Branch
Houston—University of Texas, M.D. Anderson Hospital
Houston—Commercial Diving Center, 2120 Peckham Street
Houston—NASA, Manned Space Center, Physiological Training Branch
Pasadena—J And J Marine
Brooks Air Force Base—US Air Force School of Aerospace Medicine
San Antonio—Southwest Research Institute
UTAH
Salt Lake City—St. Mark's Hospital
VIRGINIA
Fort Belvoir—US Army 77th Engineer Company
Fort Eustis—US Army Transportation School
Hampton—National Aeronautics and Space Administration
Norfolk—US Naval Amphibious Base
Richmond—Medical College of Virginia
WASHINGTON
Azwell—Public Utility District No.1
Bremerton—Puget Sound Naval Shipyard
Fairchild Air Force Base—US Air Force Regional Hospital
Keyport—US Naval Torpedo Station
Seattle—Providence Hospital Institute of Environmental Medicine

Seattle—Borton Divers

Seattle—Divers Institute of Technology, Inc.

Seattle—Garrison 8 Divers Corp.

Seattle—National Marine Fisheries Service

Seattle—The Swedish Hospital Medical Center

Seattle—University Hospital

Seattle—Virginia Mason Research Center

Midway— Highline Community College, Redondo Pier

WISCONSIN

Milwaukee—Saint Luke's Hospital

Milwaukee—Milwaukee County Emergency hospital

CANADA

ALBERTA

Edmonton—Divers Den, 10,550 109th Street

BRITISH COLUMBIA

Nanaimo— Fisheries Research Board of Canada

Pit Meadows—Seaboard Marine Divers and Consultants Ltd.

Vancouver—British Columbia Cancer Institute

Vancouver—Vancouver General Hospital

Vancouver—Videospection Engineering Company, Ltd.

North Vancouver—International Hydrodynamics Company, Ltd.

North Vancouver—Can Dive Services, Ltd.

Victoria—Fleet Diving Unit

MANITOBA

Winnipeg–Manitoba Cancer Treatment and Research

NEWFOUNDLAND

St. John's–Memorial University of Newfoundland

NOVA SCOTIA

Dartmouth–Bedford Institute of Oceanography

Dartmouth—Canadian Naval Fleet Diving Unit
ONTARIO
Downsview—Defense Research Establishment, Toronto
London—Ontario Cancer Foundation
Toronto—Toronto General Hospital
QUEBEC
Montreal—Royal Victoria Hospital
Pointe aux Trembles—International Underwater Contractors, Ltd.
PUERTO RICO
Caba Rojo–Marine Resources Development Foundation
San German–Hospital de la Concepción
MEXICO
Acapulco —Divers de México
Acapulco–Icacor Naval Base, Primera Compañía del Comandó Submarino
México City–Hospital de Emergencias de Coyoacán (XOCO)
México City–Centro Hospitalario "20 de Noviembre"
México City–Equipos y Técnicas, S.A., Y/O Organización Submarina Mexicana, S.A., Guterberg 47–803